Instructor's Manual

Abnormal Psychology

Second Edition

Rosenhan and Seligman

Instructor's Manual

Abnormal Psychology
Second Edition

Rosenhan and Seligman

JOSEPH LOWMAN
UNIVERSITY OF NORTH CAROLINA–CHAPEL HILL

W. W. NORTON AND COMPANY
NEW YORK   LONDON

Cover illustration: *Composition: "City People"*
by Abraham Rattner. Collection of Charles E. Curry.
Photograph courtesy of Kennedy Galleries, Inc., New York.

ISBN 0-393-95700-4

W. W. Norton & Company, Inc., 500 Fifth Avenue, New York, N.Y. 10110
W. W. Norton & Company Ltd., 37 Great Russell Street, London WC1B 3NU

1 2 3 4 5 6 7 8 9 0

Contents

Instructor's Manual

Abnormal Psychology

Second Edition

Rosenhan and Seligman

Teaching the Abnormal Psychology Course

The aim of this manual is to aid instructors who teach abnormal psychology courses ranging in size from fifteen to several hundred students. Most of us who follow the traditional lecture/discussion format will find success with the course if we take the time to plan lectures and individual class meetings creatively and if we deliver them skillfully. The model underlying the suggestions in this manual was based on educational research about college classrooms and an informal study of a group of "master teachers" (*Mastering the Techniques of Teaching*, Lowman, 1984). College classrooms are dramatic and interpersonal arenas before they are settings for intellectual discourse and learning. To teach content effectively, an instructor must be able to present material clearly and in ways that engage students' attention. The most successful instructors, especially in smaller classes and with less mature students, will *also* be those who are interpersonally skilled, who understand the psychology of students and classroom groups well, and who are able to foster rapport, independence, and motivation.

This section presents an overview of teaching skills as applied to the abnormal psychology course. The use of *SuperShrink*, a computer interview simulation, as an out-of-class laboratory, is also described. Subsequent sections present, for each chapter in the Rosenhan and Seligman text, an overall perspective, a sample lecture outline containing major points and appropriately placed discussion queries, a description of classroom demonstrations instructors may want to use, annotated supplemental readings and films, and identification, short-answer, and essay questions.

Initial Attitudes

Every student taking a course in abnormal psychology comes with positive expectations and a number of specific questions they hope to have answered. Some have immediate concerns about their own emotional problems or the troubling behavior of family members or friends. Others will be most concerned about the past, about psychopathology they have experienced or encountered in another. Still others may be fascinated by unusual human behavior and eager to learn about those showing it. In short, most students come to this course motivated to learn about abnormal psychology. Because of this, it is difficult for us to teach this course badly!

Course Goals

Most instructors will have goals as to what they believe their students should learn from the course. First, students should learn a number of *facts* about psychopathology. They should be able to describe the major diagnostic categories in DSM-III-R, be able to make rough distinctions among them, even when applied to specific case examples, know the major theories of causation and supporting research, and be familiar with the major treatment approaches. Second, the course should help students to increase their *thinking skills*. Students should be able to critically evaluate evidence supporting various theories or therapeutic interventions and to integrate their personal experiences with research findings. Third, some instructors may also desire to change students' *attitudes* about abnormality. They may want students to see persons showing psychopathology as much more like themselves than different and as needing understanding, tolerance, and concern. Such instructors will be educating students to be informed and concerned citizens. Finally, for some instructors, the abnormal psychology course will have the additional goal of giving students *guidance* in overcoming problems and living emotionally healthy lives.

A textbook can do only so much toward meeting these goals. If the course is to be of highest quality, class meetings should be such that students look forward to coming to them. The most successful classroom instructors will do far more than rehash what is presented in the text. They will bring the perspective of experienced clinicians and researchers to selected topics and case studies, focus the group's attention on critical or controversial issues, and stimulate their students' thinking and imagination through lectures, discussion, demonstrations, and field trips, so that the students can see the relevance of the course to their own lives. As much as anything else, though, the best courses will be those in which the instructor is enthusiastic about the subject and eager to share his or her knowledge with students. Although college students learn from engaging and stimulating teachers even if the teachers are cold and distant, most will be *more* motivated to learn from instructors who are warm and approachable, in addition to being interesting (Keaveny and McGann, 1978; Marques, Lane, and Dorfman, 1979; Uranowitz and Doyle, 1980). Teachers who show personal interest in students— learning their names during the first few classes is an excellent way to begin —make it more likely that students will apply their energies and intellectual talents to learning what they have to teach them. Effort spent pursuing interpersonal goals is more than repaid by producing enjoyable classes to teach as well as increased learning and satisfaction among students.

Specific Teaching Skills

PLANNING

The abnormal psychology course is similar to the introductory psychology course in that there is "so much to present, so little time." We are all faced with decisions about what to leave out of class presentations or to touch on only lightly. So in organizing a course, one place to begin is with what we want students to know when the course is over. Whether one jots down a few general goals or prepares a list of formal learning objectives, a few minutes of overall planning will help make easier the decisions about what to cover in depth.

One of the most important decisions has already been made: the choice of text. All abnormal psychology texts begin with general considerations before covering specific diagnostic categories and treatment approaches. The initial chapters in this text cover the various models of psychopathology and in so doing provide a solid basis for the subsequent chapters on specific categories and interventions. The order in which Rosenhan and Seligman have presented various topics is logical and consistent with their theoretical emphases. Critical themes and issues reappear in increasing detail. Following their structure will make things simpler for everyone. Let the Rosenhan and Seligman text provide the core content of your course and enrich it by the inclusion of other assignments and experiences consistent with your own experiences and biases.

In deciding how many classes to devote to each chapter, how much supplemental reading (if any) to assign or review in class, whether to assign written work, and what films or field trips to schedule, be guided by *reality* (there are only so many class meetings) and the need to build in *interest* and an occasional *change of pace* for students. Varying class format every three or four meetings will keep things from becoming too predictable. Scheduling exams first and fitting chapter topics to the time between them distributes work load better than scheduling exams mainly on logical organization of topics. Some instructors have benefited by leaving an unscheduled class meeting before each exam as an "expansion joint." Also reserving a class meeting or two at the end of the term will allow time to put the course into perspective and help students integrate the considerable information that has been covered.

The next task is to plan individual class meetings. Think of these as "artistic wholes" needing an engaging beginning, a gradual buildup of suspense, and a decisive ending. If at all possible, plan material that can be completed in one session. Including occasional case examples, discussion questions or issues, and classroom demonstrations will help students relax a bit, and increase their involvement. The sample lecture outlines suggested in this manual have been prepared with these considerations in mind.

LECTURES

Though lectures are one of the least effective methods of conveying information (Thompson, 1974; Bowman, 1979) and no longer serve their original purpose—to transmit information to students' notes—they have a number of important functions. Lectures are useful for emphasizing organization and critical points, clarifying difficult issues, and inspiring students to appreciate the importance of what they read in texts. To be sure, at their worst lectures are simply awful, but at their best they are magnificent!

Other than a thorough grasp of the subject, the most essential lecturing skill is the ability to speak well before groups: to project articulately and to convey a feeling of immediacy and spontaneity, even when the lecture has been carefully prepared beforehand. Good delivery is an essential ingredient to a fine lecture.

When selecting points to be made, avoid trying to cover everything. It simply cannot be done. Present instead points that are of central importance, special difficulty, or of high interest to students. Students will only be able to absorb four or five points in a single class (McKeachie, 1978), so choose them wisely.

After briefly connecting the day's class to previous meetings, begin with a question, paradox, or short case description to capture students' interest at the outset. They are more likely to pay full attention to more theoretical or technical topics if a positive anticipation is created early on. Good lectures also have variety. The instructor can break up the presentation every ten to fifteen minutes with a discussion query, a humorous comment or observation, or an illustrative anecdote. Case illustrations (especially of patients you have seen yourself) are an especially effective way to break the routine. Remember that the responsibility for presenting content lies chiefly with the text; the purposes of the class meetings are to captivate, to illustrate, and to motivate.

Organization and involvement can be enhanced by the use of audiovisual aids. Overhead transparencies, 35 mm slides, and videotape or film clips can effectively capture students' attention (especially in large classes with over 100 students), as well as emphasizing organization and demonstrating patient behaviors and treatment or research methods. Such electronic devices do have drawbacks (they require advance planning, take time to set up for use, and sometimes fail to work properly), however, and are no substitute for content well selected and delivered. A skillful lecturer can usually get along fine without them by using blackboards or flipcharts. Although neither necessary nor sufficient, audiovisual aids can enrich lectures greatly.

DISCUSSION

Like the lecture, discussion at its worst is painful for students and instructor alike. For this reason, or because they see it as wasting time that could be better spent presenting information, many teachers avoid using it. Yet, when used skillfully for appropriate purposes, discussion can increase involvement, promote rapport, and encourage independent thinking.

As McKeachie (1978) notes, "discussion is probably not effective for presenting new information which the student is already motivated to learn" (p. 35). Discussion has been shown to be the best way of helping students assimilate and integrate what they hear in lecture or read on their own. It is also a good way to encourage students to question the value assumptions they make about the emotionally disturbed and to apply the course to their own experiences. Pausing for discussion occasionally also gives everyone (the instructor included) a chance to catch a breath and increases involvement in what follows. Much of the content of the abnormal psychology course is provocative and, if an instructor wishes to change students' attitudes as well as increasing their factual knowledge, some class time should be devoted to giving students a chance to respond.

Using discussion well involves far more than asking, "Any questions?" or "What do others think?" It is more likely to be successful if the questions asked are focused. For example, students can be asked to identify with the patients under study ("If your mood was that low and you felt that hopeless, how might you view the prospect of dying?"), to compare and contrast topics ("How are the behavioral and cognitive ways of viewing abnormality similar?"), or to consider their own attitudes and behavior toward unusual persons ("What is your initial reaction when you meet someone socially who is particularly unattractive, dominating, or shy?"). Students are more likely to become involved in discussion if it seems *mutual*, that is, if the instructor seems genuinely puzzled by the question he or she proposes. Avoid recitation, asking students to answer factual questions about content in the readings ("According to Cleckley, what are the characteristics of antisocial personalities?"). For students to feel comfortable discussing, it is critical that they be given as much freedom to be wrong as possible. To do this, qualify queries by using words like "might," "could," and "your" to emphasize that it is the students' personal thoughts and attitudes that are of interest. Students are more likely to respond to "What does psychoanalysis mean to you?" or "Are you a Freudian?" than to "What is psychoanalysis?"

For many instructors, the hardest part of using discussion is getting it started. Posing a brief query will make students more likely to respond, but waiting for ten seconds or so before rephrasing the query and asking it again will also help condition the class to discussion. Although the silence can seem interminable, do not give up easily, especially by calling on a student who has not indicated he or she wishes to speak. Also avoid giving a mini-lecture following the first comment. Others will speak if given a chance.

Students are more likely to want to speak if aroused by a common emotional experience or presented with a provocative query—and it is clear the teacher expects them to respond.

Students are also more likely to speak if they are reinforced rather than punished. Positive nonverbal messages such as smiles and nods are reinforcing for most students. Stressing the insightful or creative aspects of each comment can also be useful. Avoid interrogating students about their comments unless it is well into the term (when students are likely to be less anxious about evaluation) or unless the student is a frequent contributor.

Students will tire of discussion after five or six comments; instructors should then redirect, integrate, and summarize before posing another query or resuming lecture. Discussion should be guided gently with a pleasantly inquisitive air. Playing devil's advocate can also promote student thought if done warmly and with a smile. Because leading discussion requires considerable teacher spontaneity (to a great extent, instructors must "let" discussion happen), a sensitive sense of timing, and well-honed communication skills, many experienced teachers believe that leading a first-rate discussion is more difficult than presenting an outstanding lecture (Eble, 1976).

There is nothing inherently desirable about students speaking in class. But when used appropriately to promote involvement, thinking, and rapport, discussion can enrich a course greatly and increase what students will learn from it.

ASSIGNING WORK

Reading. Two major types of supplemental reading assignments can be made to increase students' involvement and give them an opportunity to apply what they are learning about psychopathology. The first of these consist of book-length case studies of persons showing various types of abnormality. Students can be assigned one of these to read and criticize as part of a term-paper requirement or essay on the final exam. The second type of reading may include specific articles from *Psychology Today* or from the research literature, or from the *Casebook and Study Guide*, by Christopher Peterson of the University of Michigan, Ann Arbor, which was designed specifically to accompany the second edition of Rosenhan and Seligman's text. Specific articles are suggested in the chapter discussions that appear later in this manual. The following are suggestions of longer works that can be assigned to be read over the term.

Rokeach, M. (1964). *The three Christs of Ypsilanti*, New York: Knopf. This is a classic account of the effects of putting three paranoid schizophrenics, each of whom believed he was Jesus Christ, into intimate contact with each other. Rokeach presents detailed case histories of the three men before he assembled them at the Ypsilanti State Hospital. His book follows the three patients and the changes in their delusions and behavior which occurred during the years he studied them. This book illustrates vividly the delusional thought disorder shown by many paranoid schizophrenics. Students will become increasingly able to correctly interpret the men's confusing and highly symbolic speech to Rokeach and one another. Students will come to see the men as unique persons much like themselves rather than as abstractions or "weirdos." Because some of the interventions Rokeach attempted would no longer be allowed in our age of concern about patients' rights, this work will also raise important ethical issues about research and treatment.

Plath, Sylvia. (1981). *The bell jar*. New York: Bantam Windstone. This is a semiautobiographical novel about a talented and sensitive young writer who becomes depressed and suicidal late in her college career. The novel explores in depth the hopelessness of depression and the attendant cognitive distortions that characterize the depressed individual's experience. Written in the first person, the book permits students to gain an understanding of Esther's world from the inside out. Issues raised in the book include the role of childhood bereavement in adult depression and suicide-prone behavior, the potential hazards and benefits of electroshock therapy, and the many paradoxes of neurotic functioning. Students frequently relate well to the character because they are facing the same developmental tasks as those confronted by Esther: career choice, heterosexual intimacy, and so forth.

Keyes, Daniel. (1982). *The minds of Billy Milligan*. New York: Bantam Books. In a landmark trial in 1977, William Stanley Milligan was acquitted of charges of rape and kidnapping by reason of insanity caused by multiple personality—the first such court decision in history. This book is an extremely well-written, factual history of the life of Billy Milligan, who was tormented by twenty-four distinct personalities. The family of characters included many men, three female personalities, and several children, all of whom fought for control of Billy's consciousness. As the horrific events of Billy's childhood are recounted, students gain key insights into the pathogenic potential of physical and sexual abuse and the structure of neurotic conflict. Additionally, the book follows Billy after his trial when he was put in a maximum security hospital for the criminally insane. At that time the successful fusion of the twenty-four personalities was undone due to unfavorable press coverage of the case. This book is remarkable and absorbing and will stimulate students to debate the issues of legal responsibility and mental illness, leaving no doubt as to the validity of the multiple personality syndrome, however rare its occurrence.

Hinckley, Jack, & Hinckley, Joan. (1985). *Breaking Points*. East Rutherford, NJ: Berkley. John Hinckley's parents' account of their son's life up until and after attempting to assassinate President Ronald Reagan is both interesting and moving. Students will find that this book provides an illustrative case history of violent behavior that raises important questions about civil liberties and mental health care in our society.

Axline, Virginia. (1964). *Dibs in search of self*. New York: Ballantine Books. This is the well-known story of a little boy named Dibs who discovers himself with the patient help of Virginia Axline, an authority on the technique of play therapy. Dibs is profoundly disturbed and isolated, the first son of a professional couple that rejected him from the time of his conception because of the disruption he created in their lives. He would not talk, he would not play with other children, and many suspected him of being retarded. The book summarizes his treatment with Dr. Axline and tracks his growth back toward health. Students will be greatly impressed with the power of Axline's deceptively simple techniques of nondirective play therapy. They will be awestruck at the complexity and sophistication of this young boy and will see, often for the first time, the richness of the symbolism and meaning that *is* children's play.

Greenberg, Joanna (as Hannah Green). (1964). *I never promised you a rose garden*, New York: Holt, Rinehart and Winston, Inc. This is the story of a sixteen-year-old girl who retreats into the delusional "Kingdom of Yr" and her enormous struggle to give it up and return to the real world. Although profoundly disturbed for many years, a suicide attempt prompted her commitment to a mental hospital, where three years of intensive treatment were required to untangle her from a seductive but frightening world of madness. The novel reveals many truths about the inner world of the young psychotic and the complex culture of the mental hospital. Students will gain tremendous insights into the order and meaning of the disordered experience of the schizophrenic.

Leon, G. R. (1977). *Case histories of deviant behavior: An interactional perspective* (2nd ed.). Boston: Holbrook Press.

Spitzer, R. L., Skodd, A. E., Gibbon, M., & Williams, J. B. W. (1983). *Psychopathology: A case book*. New York: McGraw-Hill.

Besides the casebook that accompanies this text, these are two other sources of short case histories of individuals showing various forms of psychopathology. Selected cases can be introduced into class presentations or assigned to students. Such readings can be assigned over an entire semester, or when relevant to specific chapters.

Computer Laboratory.   The ready availability of microcomputers on most campuses and the software package *SuperShrink* (Lowman, 1987) has made it possible to assign a computer laboratory in clinical interviewing and case formulation in lieu of papers about written case histories. *SuperShrink* is an in-depth study of a single individual (a second case will be available soon) whom students interview via microcomputers — students are the interviewers and the computers are the clients. Students then analyze the client in written reports that serve as term papers. Most students take from five to eight hours to complete each interview on the computer and to collect information and observations, which they write down in the Interviewing Workbook for use in their written reports. Students report greatly enjoying the *SuperShrink* experience and learning a great deal from the challenge of applying psycho-dynamic and cognitive-behavioral principles to the complex information gathered.

Writing. All of us vary in the amount of written work we assign. Common reasons for assigning papers are to help students to hone their writing skills, to learn how to survey the research literature, to encourage independent reading and thinking, to apply course concepts to specific examples, or to promote critical evaluation of research. Regardless of the specific objective, it is better to limit somewhat students' choice of topic. Asking students to write a paper on "a specific diagnostic category or therapeutic method of your choice" is more likely to fit an instructor's objectives than assigning a paper on "whatever topic you wish." A good option for many purposes is to assign a single reading assignment to the whole class (*The Three Christs of Ypsilanti*, for example) and to ask them to apply whatever course topic they wish to it. Letting them choose books to read and write about from the list discussed previously also works well.

The greatest drawbacks to written assignments are administrative, and these can be offset by skillful handling of the assignment by the instructor. Their length is of less importance than the objectives a college teacher has for them. Requesting papers to be turned in two or three weeks before the end of the term allows sufficient time to grade and return them before classes are over. Students can also be encouraged to rewrite their papers and resubmit them for a second grading. Grading papers blindly will prevent your knowledge of how students have done on other work from influencing their grades on the paper. This will also emphasize the fact that it is their work, not themselves, that is being judged. Getting papers to be submitted on time can be particularly frustrating, especially if "cops and robbers" punishments are stressed for late papers. Simply announcing a due date, stressing that it was chosen to allow enough time for the papers to be evaluated closely, and that papers will be returned promptly with specific feedback written on them usually suffices to bring most of them in near the desired date. Some students will always be a few days late, but the control issue around the deadline will be diffused for instructor and students alike.

Field Trips. If a picture is worth a thousand words, then a field trip in an abnormal psychology course is worth a thousand 35 mm slides. Few experiences can do more to add to what has been learned about psycho-pathology from reading and class attendance than a trip to a psychiatric hospital or mental retardation center. Although every student may not have a flexible-enough schedule to attend, organize a trip for those who can and, if at all possible, go along yourself. Not only will you have many opportunities to teach students about what they will be seeing, the time spent together will promote rapport with those who go.

Students can also be encouraged to take advantage on their own of other opportunities for contact with persons showing difficulties in living. Some schools have organized volunteer programs allowing students to make regular visits to psychiatric or mental retardation institutions, nursing homes, or prisons, or to have direct contact with children as tutors or "big brothers or sisters." Although students should not be given extra credit for such experiences, allowing students to include what they have learned in written assignments or essays is appropriate.

EVALUATING STUDENT WORK

Evaluating students and assigning grades is for many the most unpleasant part of college teaching; a considerable mythology surrounds these practices. Some instructors believe that students will not be motivated to learn unless graded severely; others believe quite the opposite—that students will not be able to do more than memorize details unless given considerable freedom to pursue learning and to be evaluated generously. Still others believe that hard grading and student satisfaction are inversely correlated, that instructors who are demanding will not receive high ratings of their teaching from students. In fact, research indicates that *none* of these beliefs is correct (Lowman, 1984; Milton, Pollio, and Eisen, 1986). The fact that belief in them persists reveals that evaluation is an emotional issue for faculty as well as for students.

A major purpose of this instructors' manual is to aid the evaluation process. For each chapter in the text, identification, short-answer, and essay test items are included. In addition, the test item file that accompanies the text contains nearly a thousand multiple-choice questions. Choosing evaluation methods that judge students fairly and assess what you have tried to teach them is much more complex, however, than simply giving this manual or the test item file to a secretary and asking him or her to select items from those provided.

The first consideration in selecting or constructing evaluation methods is their purpose. Are the exams more to see if all students mastered the basic content or to spread students out along a distribution—to see how *much* some of them learned? An exam of the first type will be easier for everyone, but it may not motivate brighter students as would a more challenging exam. Are the exams to assess how well students memorized details from the text and lectures or to see how well they can apply the concepts to examples or can demonstrate sophisticated thinking by critiquing theories or hypotheses? Some testing methods are better for some objectives than others.

Regardless of objectives, however, practical issues must also be considered. Are 20 or 200 students to be assessed? Is there a teaching assistant to help with grading? Are exams given in fifty or seventy-five-minute class hours or in longer sessions scheduled by the college or university? Are regular exams during a term traditional in your setting or do most instructors use papers, "take-homes," or a large final at the end?

It is possible to select evaluation methods from those provided in this manual that will produce comparative data reflecting fairly the learning differences among students as well as motivating them to learn. This is best accomplished by mixing testing strategies, avoiding trickery and triviality, using items of varying difficulty, and giving students specific guidance on how to study beforehand. Advantages and disadvantages of each of the item types included here are as follows.

Multiple-Choice Items.   The multiple-choice items in the test item file have been carefully constructed and screened to ensure that they are clear, that they reflect important content, and that students are frequently required to demonstrate understanding and thinking in addition to memorization. Feel free to modify them if you wish but be careful to avoid introducing ambiguity or unnecessary difficulty. These items can be scored quickly (use a computer-scoring service if one is available) and analyzed statistically to produce comparative data on item difficulty and mathematical power to distinguish students in the top and bottom parts of the class based on total scores. Although these items are easier than short-answer or essay items (Gronlund, 1982), students will focus on details when studying for them (Milton, 1978).

Short-Answer and Identification Items.   These items are much easier to construct, but they take considerably longer to grade than multiple-choice items. Their advantage is that they can focus on details as much as multiple-choice items, but they can also be used to assess thinking. Students can be asked to compare and contrast specific concepts as well as to give definitions, for example. To ensure that they are scored objectively, write out answers to each question and use them as models to decide how much credit to give students' answers. Even if these items are not used exclusively, several can be easily added to multiple-choice exams.

Reverse IDs.   The objectives of reverse IDs are similar to those of short-answer and identification questions, but this type of item is much easier and faster to grade. Include on your exams a series of definitions of important course terms — garnered from the glossary list at the back of the text — and ask students to write the appropriate name in a blank beside the definition. Giving students a list of important items beforehand and telling them where definitions may be found guides their study and helps reduce anxiety about this type of question.

Essays.   Broad, integrative essays are ideal at the end of a course when the objective is to encourage students to pull together what they have learned and form their own opinions about key issues (the relative utility of psychoanalytic, behavioral, cognitive, humanistic, and biomedical models, for example). They are easy to construct but exceedingly difficult to grade reliably and fairly. Unlike short answers, model answers cannot be constructed. Some instructors choose particular student papers as models, however, and use them to typify "A," "B," "C," and "D" papers. Giving the same amount of attention to each paper is the most difficult part of grading essays. Avoid grading very many in one sitting, and spread them out over several days if at all possible.

Although evaluation is one of the least satisfying parts of college teaching, planning carefully the methods to be used and applying them with fairness and concern for students can minimize its negative aspects and maximize the positive motivational effect it has on learning. The evaluation materials presented in this manual have been constructed with these ends in mind.

Why Try to Excel in the Classroom?

The abnormal psychology course offers tremendous potential for being one of the most intellectually provocative and personally satisfying courses students will take in their college career. By examining persons living at the fringes of the human condition, a powerful mirror is held up to reflect light on common characteristics and psychological processes in all of us. Offering a course as advocated here clearly takes energy, effort, and talent. A relevant question to close this section is, "Why should an instructor try to excel in the classroom?"

If making tenure is all that matters, energy put into attaining excellence in teaching is probably misplaced. Many excellent researchers are also excellent teachers, but avoiding research to concentrate on classroom excellence is not a good survival strategy at many institutions. Similarly, striving for excellence in this area to achieve recognition from colleagues or awards is unlikely to be ultimately satisfying.

The interviews upon which I based the model of effective teaching, however, convinced me that most outstanding classroom teachers make the effort to excel because of more personal reasons. For some of them, it is out of commitment to the future of their discipline. They hope to attract and nurture the students with the most talent. For others, it is because they find "giving away what they know" and personal relationships with students immensely satisfying. Most of the men and women I interviewed were motivated to excel in the classroom, however, because they found it inherently satisfying to captivate, to inspire, and to motivate students to work hard to master their subject.

I hope the ideas in this manual prove useful to your efforts to offer your students an introductory survey of this fascinating topic.

References

Bowman, J. S. (1979). Lecture-discussion format revisited. *Improving College and University Teaching, 27,* 25–27.

Eble, K. (1988). *The craft of teaching: Mastering the professor's art* (2nd ed.). San Francisco: Jossey-Bass.

Gronlund, N. E. (1982). *Constructing achievement tests* (3rd ed.). Englewood Cliffs, NJ: Prentice-Hall.

Keaveny, T. J., & McGann, A. F. (1978). Behavioral dimensions associated with students' global ratings of college professors. *Research in Higher Education, 9,* 333–345.

Lowman, J. (1984). *Mastering the techniques of teaching.* San Francisco: Jossey-Bass.

Lowman, J. (1987). *SuperShrink.* San Diego, CA: Harcourt Brace Jovanovich.

McKeachie, W. J. (1986). *Teaching tips: A guidebook for the beginning college teacher* (8th ed.). Lexington, MA: Heath.

Marques, T. E., Lane, D. M., & Dorfman, P. W. (1979). Toward the development of a system for instructional evaluation: Is there consensus regarding what constitutes effective teaching? *Journal of Educational Psychology, 71,* 840–849.

Milton, O. (1978). Classroom testing. In O. Milton et al., *On college teaching: A guide to contemporary practices.* San Francisco: Jossey-Bass.

Milton, O., Pollio, H. R., & Eisen, J. A. (1986). *Making sense of college grades: Why the grading system does not work and what can be done about it.* San Francisco: Jossey-Bass.

Thompson, R. (1974). Legitimate lecturing. *Improving College and University Teaching, 22,* 163–164.

Uranowitz, S. W., & Doyle, K. O. (1980). Being liked and teaching: The effects and bases of personal likability in college instruction. *Research in Higher Education, 9,* 15–41.

CHAPTER 1

The Meanings of Abnormality

Overview

It is common practice to devote the first class to administrative concerns with little or no coverage of content. Even in such a case it is advisable to give a brief preview of the forms of psychopathology and therapeutic methods that will be covered in the course, in addition to outlining requirements and policies. Pique students' curiosity and support their hope that this course will answer personal as well as intellectual questions about the nature of abnormality. The first meeting is also a good place to warn them about "interns' syndrome" and to stress that although it can cause personal anxiety, it can also give them empathic insights into the human beings they will be studying.

Most instructors will consider Chapter 1 in the second class meeting. The overall objective for Chapter 1 should be to sensitize students to the many ways to answer the question, "What is abnormal and what is normal?" In answering, the ultimate dependence on relatively subjective individual judgments should be stressed. This first class is more *attitudinal* than *factual*, and the sample lecture outline reflects this by the inclusion of several discussion queries. The introductory points to be made lend themselves well to discussion, to stimulating students to become aware of their implicit assumptions about abnormality. When this class is over, students should be struck by the complexity of the question, "What is abnormality?"

Sample Lecture Outline

These introductory issues are important to the more specific topics that follow and are well worth spending a whole class meeting on. Because they are attitudinal, students will have a lot to say about them, and they are thus ideal for stimulating students to consider their own thoughts, values, and observations about human nature and to share them with others when asked to do so.

1. After a brief preview of the day's topic, ask students what they think about Joyce Brown, the homeless person described in the first pages of the text: "Is this person abnormal, and if so, why do you think so?" After briefly summarizing each comment on the board, gently question its sufficiency ("So that's the only reason the person is abnormal?"), to tease out as many of the criteria presented in the book as possible.

2. After ten to fifteen minutes of discussion on this topic, list the criteria (suffering, maladaptiveness, and so on) one at a time on the board, comment on each briefly, and ask students to give examples of persons or behaviors that illustrate it. After every few topics ask, "Any questions about these so far?" The distinction between "individual well-being" and "well-being of society" is one worth commenting on, pointing out how various forms of psychopathology will emphasize one of these more than the other.

3. This discussion and presentation should have taken most of the class session. Still, try to take a few minutes to comment briefly on the issue of diagnosis. Emphasize the "family resemblance" metaphor used in the text and the hazards associated with its use.

4. Depending on how much time was spent on the nature of abnormality, there may not be enough time to treat the issue of normality in detail. If so, simply summarize the criteria of optimal living (positive attitudes about self, growth, and development, and so forth). If there are at least ten minutes remaining, ask "How can we go beyond the unsatisfying definition of normality as simply the absence of abnormality and define 'optimal living'?"

Demonstrations

1. To stimulate discussion, bring in a "pseudo-psychiatric patient" and interview him for ten to fifteen minutes. Be vague initially as to whether the person is actually a patient, but be honest afterward if someone asks about this. Have a colleague or experienced student role play a person with symptoms of a major diagnostic category and interview him briefly about his life and present symptoms. When the "patient" has left the room, ask the class, "Is this person abnormal and why do you or do you not think so?" A more deceptive version of this exercise is to have a confederate act like an angry and confused student who thinks he or she is in a religion course. Have the stooge become belligerent toward the instructor before finally leaving. Although this technique will definitely capture the class's attention—unless it has been used in other campus psychology courses recently—it is less likely to teach as much about psychopathology as an interview situation. A film clip or videotape segment showing unusual behavior or an interview with a patient can also be used for the same purpose (see the film section that follows for suggestions).

2. You might encourage students to look for an instance of abnormality around town or campus and to report on it briefly at the beginning of the next class. Many students will take this seriously, and some will bring in vivid examples to share. Such an exercise should sensitize students to notice more carefully the examples of human behavior they encounter. Encouraging rather than requiring students to do this will communicate the expectancy that they can learn outside of what is required or graded. Reserve five to ten minutes at the beginning of the next class for a few students to share their experiences and observations.

Supplemental Readings

Szasz, T. (1960). The myth of mental illness. *American Psychologist, 15,* 113—118. This classic article provides a provocative and relevant discussion of this chapter's subject. It is short, lively, and a good critique of the medical model that most students believe in implicitly when they begin the course.

Films

Abnormal psychology (26 minutes, CRM/McGraw-Hill Films, P.O. Box 641, Del Mar, CA 92014). This film provides a good overview of the course, dealing with the influences of early experiences on later psychopathology, the role of anxiety in neurosis, and illustrations of psychosis using footage of schizophrenics in a mental hospital. There is even a scene of an ECT treatment. This film can be shown outside of class in its entirety or selected scenes can be used to provoke discussion about what constitutes abnormality.

The Jolo serpent handlers (40 minutes, Karen Kramer Films, New Day Films, P.O. Box 315, Franklin Lakes, NJ 07417). This film presents vivid scenes of a snake-handling religious community in West Virginia and includes interviews with individuals about why they engage in this highly unusual and dangerous activity. One segment shows the followers singing and playing around the bed of a man as he recovers without medical treatment from a rattlesnake bite. Many segments of this film could be used to create film clips to provoke class discussion.

Examination Items

IDENTIFICATION AND SHORT-ANSWER QUESTIONS
1. What does it mean to say something is a *necessary* condition of abnormality?
2. In contrast, what is a *sufficient* condition?
3. What is iatrogenic illness?

Each of the following elements or properties of abnormality make good ID questions. Select two or three to include on the exam.

4. suffering
5. maladaptiveness
6. irrationality and incomprehensibility
7. unpredictability and loss of control
8. vividness and unconventionality
9. observer discomfort
10. violation of moral and ideal standards

The areas in which "optimality" can be recognized can be focused on in a single essay or in separate ID questions. For IDs, select two or three of the following:

11. positive attitudes about self
12. growth and development
13. autonomy
14. accurate perception of reality
15. environmental competence
16. positive interpersonal relations

ESSAY QUESTIONS

1. Give a short case description and ask students to use various elements of abnormality to answer the question, "Is the individual abnormal?"
2. Compare and contrast the "individual well-being" and "well-being of society" perspectives on maladjustment.
3. Discuss various dangers associated with applying diagnostic categories to individuals.
4. Discuss how "optimal living" can be defined.

CHAPTER 2

Abnormality across Time and Place

Overview

The ways in which people define and treat abnormality have always followed the general philosophical and social conceptions of their time and culture. This observation helps students appreciate that what they will be learning about psychopathology during the course is *also* bound up in our prevailing views of human nature, science, and society.

The historical material in this chapter is presented in a straightforward manner. Thus, there is less that needs emphasis or illustration than in the three chapters on the major models of abnormality. Given the wealth of information on more complex topics that must be covered before the end of the course, one option is to assign Chapters 1 and 2 for the same class and to spend most of the meeting on the introductory issues raised in Chapter 1. Little class time need be devoted to the material introduced in Chapter 2, other than answering whatever questions students may raise. Nonetheless, the sample chapter outline provided assumes an entire class will be spent on Chapter 2. In contrast to the content of Chapter 1, this chapter does not lend itself well to discussion, other than to answer questions and help students see that historical beliefs and practices "make sense" given how people view themselves and the world around them.

Sample Lecture Outline

1. Begin with a provocative statement like, "It is just as legitimate for an uneducated person in Mississippi to consult a "root doctor" when troubled by thoughts or behavior as for a person on New York's Park Avenue to make an appointment with a psychotherapist." Ask students to indicate how much they agree or disagree with this statement. Indicate that today's class will present information relevant to this statement.

2. Emphasize the point that general views about why certain individuals behave in unusual ways have varied throughout Western history. These general views have paralleled accepted world views: demons were thought to be the cause during times when there was a strong belief in animism; more scientific explanations became common only when rational, scientific methods became the dominant societal assumptions. Accepted methods of dealing with the abnormal have also followed general world views.

3. Focus on some of the "horror stories" of how people have been treated because of unusual behavior. Everyone has heard of the persecution of witches, but students may not realize that the great periods of persecution were not at the height but during the waning decades of the medieval period. The text cites dramatic statistics to make this clear, figures worth emphasizing in class. Although students are likely to be most interested in the origins of the psychological approach, especially Mesmer's and Charcot's work with hypnosis, the history of this topic can be delayed a few meetings and covered when the psychodynamic approach is discussed. The history of the psychiatric hospital is of more importance here. Stress that hospitals began for essentially economic reasons (to rid city streets of large masses of poor and displaced persons) and that the ideology of the French Revolution led Pinel to remove the chains from psychiatric patients. The descriptions of the treatment of the mentally disturbed in the public hospitals of Paris and London are particularly graphic and will stick in students' minds whether you mention them or not. The humanistic approach of "moral therapy" in the early nineteenth century is well worth stressing because it is so similar in method and effectiveness to contemporary nonpharmacological inpatient practices. This brief historical treatment does not cover the rise of the medical model and the biomedical hypothesis during the nineteenth century, nor does it discuss the socially oriented community mental health movement of the middle twentieth century. Although these come up later in the text, they can be previewed briefly here.

Supplemental Readings

Szasz, T. (1973). *The age of madness*. New York: Anchor Books, 1973. An interesting collection of brief historical descriptions of involuntarily hospitalized patients. Excerpts are included from the early days of psychiatric power (1650–1865), through the period when physicians' power grew dramatically (1865–1920), up until the modern era (after 1920). This work presents historically illuminating documents and anecdotes, which can be presented in class or assigned to students to read on their own.

Torrey, E. F. (1972). What Western psychotherapists can learn from witch-doctors. *American Journal of Orthopsychiatry, 43,* 69–76. The author reports the results of his studies of witchdoctors and shamans around the world. He concludes that they all call upon the principles that healers of all sorts—including contemporary psychologists and physicans—have long used to help others.

Rosen, G. (1975). *Madness in society: Chapters in the historical sociology of mental illness*. New York: Anchor Books. A comprehensive collection of readings comparing how the ancient world, the Middle Ages, and contemporary Western society view psychopathology.

Films

Again the stars (24 minutes, National Association of Mental Health Films, Film Library, 267 W. 28th St., New York, NY 10011). This is a portrayal of Philippe Pinel's removal of the chains of the patients at the Hôpital Général during the French Revolution. The importance of the political and social revolution in the treatment of the mentally ill is emphasized.

Examination Items

IDENTIFICATION AND SHORT-ANSWER QUESTIONS
1. Define *Malleus Maleficarum*.
2. What was the Greek view of hysteria?
3. Define "animal magnetism."
4. What was Breuer's hypothesis about "emotional catharsis"?
5. What was the York Retreat?
6. Define "moral treatment."

ESSAY QUESTIONS
1. Why were the public "hospitals" of the seventeenth century founded?
2. How did the treatment of the mentally ill in France before the French Revolution differ from that in England during the first part of the nineteenth century?

CHAPTER 3

The Biomedical Model

Overview

Most students of abnormal psychology have a strong bias against the biomedical model in favor of psychological ones. They tend to believe experience has a far greater effect on human behavior and personality than biology
and that most problems can be solved using strictly psychological means.
An important overall objective of this chapter is to help them become
familiar with the specific methods of the biomedical approach and to
appreciate the potential contribution it may make to understanding causes
and guiding treatments for many forms of psychopathology, especially the
major psychoses. This chapter's extensive case study on general paresis and
the introduction to the genetic research on schizophrenia both provide
excellent vehicles for meeting this end.

Students are more likely to accept the value of the biomedical approach if
it is stressed that *neither* the biomedical nor any of the psychological models
is sufficient, and that each works better with some disorders than with
others. If students can be persuaded that accepting the value of the biomedical model does not require them to dismiss the psychological models
they find appealing, they are more likely to take the biomedical approach
seriously. Also point out that both the psychological and biomedical models
of psychopathology have been around for centuries and continue to offer
competing explanations and therapies. When students know they will be
encountering these models throughout the course, they are also more likely
to take learning all of them seriously.

Sample Lecture Outline

This outline assumes an entire class will be spent on this model. Given that
two other models must be covered, some instructors may choose also to discuss the psychodynamic model, including psychoanalysis and the existential
approach. The environmentalist model, including both the behavioral and

cognitive approaches, will easily require a full session. Ideally, one session should be spent on each of these, but the wealth of material to be covered in the abnormal psychology course requires some topics to be touched on only briefly.

1. Before going into the biomedical model, a word needs to be said about *models*, what they are and how they aid scientific understanding and guide therapeutic methods. Few undergraduates will have a good background in philosophy of science, and all can benefit from a short lecture on how models or paradigms determine where scientists look for confirming and disconfirming data. It is especially hard for students to get away from the notion that models and theories are either right or wrong, proven or unproven, and to ask instead where they are and are not useful. Most students are unlikely to engage in relativistic thinking such as this on their own and need guidance from the instructor and a chance to ask for clarification. One way to enrich this topic is to give a summary of Thomas Kuhn's classic book, *The Structure of Scientific Revolutions*, listed under the Supplemental Readings for this chapter.

2. The meat of this chapter consists of the four illustrations of how those favoring the biomedical approach have sought causes associated with *germs, genetic links, biochemical changes*, and *neuroanatomical changes*. A good place to begin is to make the point that one first identifies a *syndrome*, or cluster of associated symptoms, then searches for an *etiology*, usually discarding numerous false leads along the way, before trying various *treatments*.

3. Focus next on the story of general paresis and how scientists came to see it as a distinct disease resulting from syphilis. A good discussion question to ask is, "Why was the link between syphilis and general paresis so difficult to establish?" Whether they have read the chapter carefully or not, students will be able to propose many problems that impeded establishing this link. Those mentioned in the text (the long time delay between initial infection and the organic psychosis, the shame associated with the disorder, and difficulties diagnosing it) are especially important to stress because they will be encountered later in attempts to understand other forms of psychopathology. In addition to any others proposed by the students, you may want to add a fourth important point to those proposed in the text: Only about 5 percent of those with untreated syphilis ever develop general paresis. Stress that the notable success with general paresis continues to give hope to biomedical researchers that many (or all) forms of major psychosis will one day be found to have a definite biomedical foundation.

4. Emphasize the relatively stable incidence of schizophrenia across different cultures and over time. Also tell students they will be learning much more about this issue later on. For now, help them to differentiate *concordant* and *discordant* percentages and to learn the basic idea of the "dopamine hypothesis." When the course is over they will be able to say a great

deal more about the genetic basis of schizophrenia and bipolar affective disorder and the biochemical or neuroanatomical basis for major psychopathology. They will also understand how various drugs used to treat schizophrenia and bipolar disorder provide support for the biomedical model. Given that the objective of this chapter is to give them an introduction to the biomedical approach, it is not necessary to go into more detail concerning these issues here.

5. As a way of concluding the discussion of this approach, ask students, "For now, how many of you favor the biomedical hypothesis over the psychological approaches? Why?" This will stimulate them to evaluate this approach and will enable you to work in the strengths and weaknesses of this model.

Supplemental Readings

Kuhn, T. (1960). *The structure of scientific revolutions*. Chicago: University of Chicago Press. This classic essay makes an analogy between scientific and political revolutions, arguing that science progresses in spurts and ebbs as competing paradigms are proposed, compete, and eventually overcome older ones. This thesis is highly relevant to the comparisons between competing paradigms that students will be making throughout the course. Although some students will have encountered this work in other courses, most will not and everyone can benefit from a short presentation of this important essay on scientific method and intellectual progress.

Sacks, O. (1987). *The man who mistook his wife for a hat and other clinical tales*. New York: Harper & Row. In this highly readable paperback collection of neurological cases, Sacks tells his stories in a way that is amusing and provocative, yet respectful and philosophical. After reading these descriptions, students are guaranteed to be impressed by the intricacies of the brain as revealed by subtle disruptions of cognitive functioning we so take for granted.

Examination Items

IDENTIFICATION AND SHORT-ANSWER QUESTIONS
1. Define "syndrome."
2. What is the first major step for a disorder to be understood as having biomedical origins?
3. Briefly describe Krafft-Ebing's critical experiment on general paresis.
4. Distinguish between "concordant" and "discordant."
5. What is the dopamine hypothesis?

ESSAY QUESTIONS
1. Why was it especially difficult to establish the link between syphilis and general paresis?
2. Given the benefit of hindsight, should Krafft-Ebing's experiment have been conducted? Why or why not?
3. Why are twins "an exquisite research tool for those who advocate the biomedical model"?
4. What are the strengths and weaknesses of the biomedical model?

CHAPTER 4

The Psychodynamic and Existential Approaches

Overview

Almost every student will come to this topic with strong initial attitudes and some prior knowledge, much of it incomplete and inaccurate. Some will come predisposed to accept uncritically anything attributed to Freud or psychoanalytic theory and others will have an equally strong aversion, perhaps saying they "don't believe in any of that Freudian nonsense." Teaching students to unlearn or expand on previous knowledge is frequently more difficult than starting from scratch.

There are many dynamic concepts and a number of theorists included in this chapter. More than one class session will likely be needed to cover the most important. In addition, numerous supplemental readings and demonstrations can be used to enrich this topic. Given that the psychodynamic approaches are of strong interest to students—even if they disavow them—and that they are still a dominant approach among many professionals and laypersons, it is appropriate to give them sufficient coverage for students to be able to evaluate them critically. Depending on how much previous coursework students will have had, relatively more or less detail need be given. No course in abnormal psychology can go into any of the theoretical approaches in much detail, so assume students will have other chances to learn more about psychodynamic theories in other courses.

Seen only as abstract concepts, psychoanalytic theory can seem overly complex, at times arbitrary, and occasionally incredible. Students are more likely to understand and appreciate the theory specifics if some of the classroom demonstrations and independent exercises suggested later are used to simulate the clinical phenomena that gave rise to them. Psychodynamic concepts did not originate in the objective and controlled atmosphere of the laboratory, but in the puzzling and unpredictable clinical setting. Helping students come face to face with the more emotional and symbolic parts of human nature will give them a more realistic basis upon which to remember and evaluate psychoanalytic theory. When you have completed this introduction to the psychodynamic approach, students should have an experiential "feel" of the rich clinical phenomena of most concern to this paradigm, as well as an objective appreciation of its scientific liabilities.

Sample Lecture Outline

1. Begin by requesting students to try to forget whatever they already know about Freud and his ideas. Urge them to consider what is said in the text and class about psychodynamic theories as if they had never heard of them before.

2. Emphasize the historical context of Freud's initial discoveries about our emotional inner life. Victorian middle-class repression of sexuality, the popularity of mechanistic notions in science during the late nineteenth century, and Freud's early wish to study neuroscience all played important roles in *how* his concepts developed.

3. Avoid simply defining and illustrating each of the many individual concepts in the chapter. Let the text define most of these. Instead, begin with a discussion of the most basic Freudian concept: the unconscious. Ask students, "How many of you believe in the unconscious?" Then ask them what evidence they use for this belief. Emphasize that each of us can on occasion recognize the presence of unusual thoughts (or dreams) that seem to reveal the workings of a usually hidden and highly emotional part of ourselves.

4. Of all the dynamic concepts presented in the chapter, those dealing with anxiety and the defense mechanisms are most relevant to students' own experience and will come up later when specific diagnostic categories are studied. Spend most of the class on them. A useful way of doing this is to give a concrete example of a college student caught in an *approach-avoidance conflict* dealing with sexual urges and moral anxiety. Create whatever details you wish, but try to make it easy for students to identify with such a student. Point out how his anxiety could come from several sources (Freud's "realistic," "neurotic," or "moral" anxiety). Then ask "How might this young man (or woman) resolve this conflict?" Students are more likely to understand the various defense mechanisms and to let you know which ones need clarification when discussing a specific situation that they can identify with. During the class discussion, list on the board the various defenses grouped according to levels of maturity. Then point out how defenses in people tend to cluster together and to be associated with various types of psychopathology: The Level I defenses (repression, delusional projection, and denial) tend to be associated with psychosis, the Level II defenses (assimilative projection) frequently result in hypochondriacal or passive-aggressive behavior, the Level III defenses (isolation, intellectualization, rationalization, and displacement) tend to be seen in many neurotics and

most of us to varying degrees, and the Level IV defenses (sublimation, conscious suppression, and impulse delay or inhibition) lead to generally positive human behaviors. Vaillant's 1977 and 1986 longitudinal studies used this system of categorizing individuals based on maturity of defenses. His studies are excellent to focus on in detail if you wish to stress longitudinal research methods.

5. Psychosexual development can be presented briefly or you can do one of the demonstrations listed in the following section. You are unlikely to manage more than this in one class meeting.

6. Discussion of the neo-Freudians alone will take most of one class session. Unless they are of major interest, however, simply answer questions about them and point out that they represent but a few of the modifications and elaborations of Freud's initial ideas that have emerged. This should help students to see psychodynamic ideas as continuing to grow even as paradigm clashes with other approaches occur.

7. Briefly present some of the modern psychodynamic theories, including self theory and existential theory. Discuss how these theories relate to and are a reaction to psychoanalytic theory. Discuss how existential theory applies the ancient philosophical issues of death anxiety, free will, and personal responsibility to psychopathology, especially to the neuroses and character disorders.

8. One of the best formulations of the role of anxiety about death in personality and psychopathology is Ernest Becker's *Denial of Death*. This classic work is too long and complex to be assigned or used to enrich lecture. The *Psychology Today* interview with Becker which is cited under the supplemental readings, however, is appropriate in length and coverage. Becker's primary ideas are as follows:

   a. Anxiety about dying underlies the anxiety over sexuality and hostility identified by Freud. Thus, psychosexual development can be reformulated as a progression in awareness of mortality.
   b. People may defend against this anxiety by believing they are "special," by avoiding dirt, anality, and sexuality because it reminds them they are animals, or by overemphasizing the importance of individual "heroics," children, careers, or wealth.

9. The text presents a detailed case study to illustrate psychoanalytic notions of both etiology and treatment methods. Spending part of one class on it or on a similarly provocative case will do much to connect the psychodynamic concepts to concrete examples. Focus on the case provided or select a "juicy" case from your own experience or one from one of the case books listed in the introduction to this manual. Present (or review) the details to the class and ask "What psychodynamic concepts do you see illustrated in this case study?"

10. Bring this model to a close by being evaluative. Ask "What are some of the positive features of this approach?" and "What are its shortcomings?" Use the student discussion to bring in and emphasize those points mentioned in the text as well as adding others of your own.

Demonstrations

1. *Free Association Demonstration.*   Students will gain a richer idea of free association as a method of uncovering emotional themes if encouraged to pay attention to their associations for a minute or so. The easiest way to do this is to ask students to write their first association to each of ten words you say. Any list of simple words ("rose," "ice," "bed") will do, but words with double, erotic, or emotional meanings (such as "prick," "slash," or "bleed") elicit more varied associations and should be mixed with more neutral ones. Wait five to ten seconds between words to allow students plenty of time to write (and edit) their initial associations. After completing the list, ask students to share what the experience was like. Some will volunteer their associations, but most will simply comment on how much longer they took to respond to some words than others or that they could see themselves avoiding initial associations they did not like. Say a word or two about Jung's origination of the word association technique (he gave a list of 100 standard words and believed differences in reaction time indicated connections to unconscious emotional themes).

Another way of demonstrating free association is to ask students to simply begin writing whatever comes into their mind for a few minutes. Suggest they avoid writing in complete sentences and feel free to simply note images or words that pop into their head. After two minutes, ask them to report on their experience. As with the word association task, some will report blocking, being unable to think of anything, and others will express surprise—even alarm—at the way their thoughts moved in a nonlogical way from association to association.

Stress that psychoanalysts and their patients spend many hours examining such associations before coming up with interpretations about what they mean. Even though you can reassure students that what they thought about in these brief demonstrations likely revealed nothing significant about their personality, you might still offer to speak with anyone individually if they have questions.

2. *Dream Log.*   Ask students to keep a dream log for a week as another way of bringing them into close contact with the complexity of their mental life. Suggest they put a notebook beside their bed and write down all their dreams immediately upon awakening for one week. Spending part of one class sharing their experiences and observations can accomplish much the same end as either of the free association exercises.

3. *Dream Analysis.* Contrast the methods of dream analysis favored by Freud and Perls by bringing in a confederate to role play a patient. Have the patient report a dream (a real or fictional one) and demonstrate Freudian analysis by having the person free associate for a few minutes to the major characters and themes in the dream. Demonstrate Gestalt analysis by having the patient act out various characters and actions. This demonstration with subsequent discussion will take about twenty minutes. The confederate may be a class student, but this demonstration requires more spontaneity and risk-taking than do most classroom demonstrations. Thus, making arrangements with a colleague or advanced student beforehand is a safer strategy.

4. *Observation of Young Children.* Students are more likely to take seriously psychodynamic notions about psychosexual development if they have first-hand experience with preschool children. If possible, set up two-hour visits for interested students to go to local preschools or simply to play with friends' preschool children. Encourage them to get involved with the children's fantasy games, following their lead as much as possible, and to note the themes of their play—aggressive, sexual, toilet.

As with the other demonstrations, students can be asked to share their experiences in class discussion. They can also be given opportunities to incorporate these experiences into written assignments if appropriate.

Supplemental Readings

Keen, S. (1974, April). The heroics of everyday life: A theorist of death confronts his own end. *Psychology Today*, 70–80. This is a very moving interview with Ernest Becker during the weeks before he died.

Hall, M. H. (1968, February). A conversation with Viktor Frankl of Vienna. *Psychology Today*, 57–63. This is a very personable interview with Viktor Frankl and Mary Hall. Frankl explains the roots of his existential theory of neurosis and psychotherapy.

Hall, M. H. (1967, December). A conversation with Carl Rogers. *Psychology Today*, 19–21. Rogers is his usual warm self in this interview. He discusses his client-centered approach to personality theory and therapy, especially its appeal and impact thus far on society.

Haley, J. (1963). Techniques of directive therapy. In J. Haley, *Strategies of psychotherapy* (pp. 41–67). New York: Grune & Stratton. In this classic chapter on the role of paradox in all psychotherapeutic methods, Haley draws on the techniques of Milton Erickson, influential hypnotherapist and intellectual inspiration for NLP, Neurolinguistic Programming, a popular therapeutic approach. Ways are outlined with which analysts and behavior therapists achieve change through relationship manipulations and paradoxical intentions.

May, R. (1970). Existential bases of psychotherapy. *American Journal of Orthopsychiatry, 30,* 685–695. May asserts that neurotic behavior is less a matter of specific symptoms than of vague general symptoms of a lack of well-being. May traces these concerns to anxiety in patients, not about sexuality or hostility, but about death. He uses a case example to illustrate how he believes many traditional Freudian concepts can be better understood within this existential framework.

Messer, S. B., & Winokur, M. (1980). Some limits to the integration of psychoanalytic and behavior therapy. *American Psychologist, 35,* 818–827. This is a "thought paper" on how the vision of life of psychoanalytic and behavior therapists are fundamentally different. In the authors' view, behavior therapists are more externally oriented and see the possibility of unambiguous happiness. Psychoanalytic therapists, in contrast, are more subjective and see the world more as a tragic and romantic place where internal conflict is accepted.

Silverman, L. H. (1976). Psychoanalytic theory: The reports of your death are greatly exaggerated. *American Psychologist, 31,* 621–637. Silverman distinguishes between "clinical" (symptoms arise from unconscious conflicts) and "metapsychological" (psychosexual development proceeds in the orderly stages Freud proposed) propositions from psychodynamic theory and presents research findings supporting major clinical propositions. He argues that the more important clinical propositions should not be dismissed because some of the metapsychological propositions have not been supported by research.

Strupp, H. H. (1972, July). Freudian analysis today. *Psychology Today,* 33–41. This leading psychoanalytically trained psychologist discusses how psychoanalysis can lead troubled persons to self-awareness, inner freedom, and maturity, while recognizing that it is not a quick or painless solution to personal or societal problems.

Whitmont, E. C. (1972, December). Jungian analysis today. *Psychology Today,* 63–72. Whitmont uses case examples to illustrate Jung's basic concepts and therapeutic techniques.

Films

Sigmund Freud: The view from within (29 minutes, University of Southern California, Division of Cinema, Film Distribution Section, University Park, Los Angeles, CA 90007). Freud's motivations to develop his theories and his life in nineteenth-century Europe are examined to provide a context for his ideas. Although not as ambitious as an excellent longer film on the same subject, *Young Dr. Freud* (Films for the Humanities, P.O. Box 2053, Princeton, NJ 08540), this short film presents important biographical information on Freud in an engaging manner.

Examination Items

IDENTIFICATION AND SHORT-ANSWER QUESTIONS

1. Define "libido."
2. Define "fixation."
3. What are "anal character traits" and why does Freud argue that "control" is an important psychological issue with roots in the anal stage?
4. Differentiate Freud's concepts of "castration anxiety" and "penis envy."
5. Define "sublimation."
6. Define "id."
7. Define "superego."
8. Define "pleasure principle."
9. What is the reality principle and how does the ego use it?
10. What are the three kinds of anxiety Freud discusses?
11. Define "core self."
12. Define "repression."
13. Differentiate between "assimilative" and "disowning" projection.
14. Define "reaction formation."
15. Define "counterphobia."
16. Define "displacement."
17. Define "identification with the aggressor."
18. Define "denial."
19. Define "isolation."
20. Define "rationalization."
21. Define "free association."
22. Define "catharsis."
23. Define "transference."
24. What is a notion of "specialness"?
25. Define "fusion."
26. Differentiate "exhortative" and "goal-directed" will.
27. Define "paradoxical intention."

ESSAY QUESTIONS

1. How does the text organize various defense mechanisms according to how effective, useful, or adaptive they are?
2. What was the basis of the disputes that led to the open break between Freud and his protégés Jung and Adler?
3. How did the beliefs of the socially oriented theorists (Sullivan, Erikson, and Fromm) differ from Freud's beliefs?
4. What are some of the positive aspects of psychodynamic theories?
5. What are some of the shortcomings of psychodynamic theories?

CHAPTER 5

The Environmentalist Model: Behavioral and Cognitive Approaches

Overview

The chapter on the environmentalist model encourages students to integrate the behavioral and cognitive models into a single perspective. Before they can do this, students must first overcome the initial resistance many of them will have to seeing the behavioral perspective sympathetically. As is true for the psychodynamic model, students are likely to have prior attitudes about the behavioral approach. Some will be quite sympathetic, but others will associate behavioral therapies with "big brother" forms of social control and cruel punishments of prisoners done in the name of treatment. The addition of cognitive phenomena to this model in recent years should increase the attractiveness to students. A first objective, then, is to persuade students to give the behavioral model a fair hearing, seeing the behavioral model as a world view with a long philosophical tradition rather than merely a collection of specific techniques or isolated abuses. Students are more likely to be able to do this if they are helped to experience first hand how the behavioral model, especially with the addition of cognitive principles, can be usefully applied to some forms of abnormal behavior. The demonstrations section describes several ways to do this.

The chapter begins with a review of basic learning concepts students will have been exposed to in previous coursework (UCS, CR, extinction, and so forth). Some will still remember them correctly, but most will not understand them well enough to appreciate fully how they can be applied to psychopathology. The sample lecture outline suggests one way of handling this dilemma, highlighting a few essential concepts while allowing students to ask questions about others.

The cognitive model is an integration of the emphasis of the psychodynamic model on internal experience and the focus of behavioral approaches on learning from association and reinforcement. An overall objective of this chapter is to show how thoughts and feelings can be critical cognitive mediators of external reinforcement contingencies. Seeing how expectations, attributions, and beliefs can influence the impact of external stimuli and responses can help students integrate their own experience with social learning concepts and research findings. Illustrations from cognitive behavior therapy can help students appreciate the practical implications of this view.

Sample Lecture Outline

1. Begin by asking: "What are your associations to behaviorism?" A short discussion on students' previous knowledge and attitudes helps set the stage for a request to seriously rethink this approach to human nature and evaluate anew its ability to suggest useful insights and interventions.

2. Set the stage for specific behavioral concepts by putting the behavioral approach into perspective. Point out that it is an heir to *associationism*, a belief in the power of experience in determining human nature, which led, among other things, to the rhetoric of the French and American revolutions. After mentioning the emphases on *environmentalism, experimentation,* and *optimism*, ask students, "What are the implications of these assumptions for how a behaviorist would view psychopathology?"

3. It is imperative that students understand the basic Pavlovian and operant paradigms and how they can be combined to explain many abnormal behaviors. Most of this class must be spent on them. One way of finding out what students remember is to present the essential format of classical conditioning (aversive stimuli paired with previously neutral ones) and then ask students to use this approach (and the specific concepts of UCS, UCR, CS, CR, and stimulus generalization) to explain how a specific symptom could have been formed. Some useful symptoms are as follows:

   a. Following the funeral of his grandfather, a seven-year-old child becomes extremely fearful of riding in cars, especially black cars.
   b. A middle-aged woman begins to feel nauseous and frequently vomits in the parking lot of the hospital when she arrives for her cancer chemotherapy.

   Following this exercise, use a similar method of reviewing the operant approach. The same symptoms can be used to show how secondary gain provides reinforcement for the avoidance behaviors of not riding in cars (to school or church) and having to delay or miss chemotherapy sessions.

4. When the case illustrations of classical and operant conditioning have been completed, write on the board (or distribute in a handout) a list of the essential learning concepts students should be familiar with. Take a few minutes to answer any questions students have about any of them and offer to meet individually with students who are still uncertain.

5. Indicate that the cognitive approach was developed by a number of behaviorists who were dissatisfied with radical behaviorism's narrow behavioral emphasis. Rather than side with Skinnerians or abandon a belief in the efficacy of learning theory to explain complex human behavior, the cognitive behaviorists chose to acknowledge the importance of thoughts and feelings but to think of them as obeying the same learning principles that control external behaviors. Stress that thoughts are not seen as epiphenomena but as essential links in [stimulus]-[cognitive mediator]-[response] connections.

6. A good way to show the complexity of expectations and attributions is to administer the abbreviated Attributional Style Scale as illustrated in the demonstrations section below. The discussion following the exercise can be guided to emphasize the independence of the internal-external, stable-unstable, and global-specific dimensions and their relationship to depressed mood in college students.

7. An alternative approach is to use the following case description of a person with self-defeating beliefs about himself and others. After describing the case illustration to the class ask, "What implicit beliefs about himself and others does this individual appear to be having?" This case can also be used to illustrate how cognitive-behavioral therapists might attempt to help this person change.

> John is a sophomore at a large Midwestern university. After he did not receive a bid from any houses at the end of fraternity rush, he was so embarrassed, disappointed, and angry that he spent most of his time in his dormitory room and missed many classes. At his roommate's insistence, he went to the clinic run by the psychology department to speak with a therapist. The following are notable things he said during the initial interview. "I can't tell you how pissed I am at those snobby Greek bastards! I mean, they really put it to me this time, really messed up my G.P.A. I guess I should have known better, I've always been a loser—never got invited to belong to the right clubs in high school, either. What hurts most is thinking those guys don't like me, think I'm such a nerd they don't want to be seen with me. I guess I must be a total reject not to be able to get even one house to be willing to take a chance on me. If I had only gotten a bid everything would have been O.K. I know I'd study harder and make better grades to keep up the image of the house. Because of all the parties I'd have learned how to be more social with girls, learned skills I can use later on in business. I feel so ashamed! I . . . I just don't want to be seen by any of those people on campus. I don't want to give them the satisfaction of seeing how bad I feel since they shafted me."

8. Bring the environmentalist model to a close by asking, "What do you think about the cognitive-behavioral approach? What are its strong and weak points as a model of abnormal psychology?"

Demonstrations

1. Using small bits of food to shape simple motor responses in hungry animals is an impressive demonstration of the power of contingent reinforcement. Bring in a laboratory animal or family pet (dog, gerbil, or hamster) that has not eaten in twenty-four hours, and use food to shape simple behaviors in the animal. Dogs can be trained to jump over a barrier and rodents can be easily shaped to rise up and walk on their hind legs—even to do back flips.

2. Use student volunteers to demonstrate stimulus gradients and the ability of symbols to elicit fear. First, ask all students to use a 1 to 10 scale to rate themselves on fear of snakes. Then request two groups of students to come forward for a harmless demonstration. Five to ten students in each group is ideal, although two or three is sufficient. Students are more likely to come up if they know they will not be forced to do anything and will not be alone. Instruct the class to note only how the subjects behave, ignoring as much as possible what they think their classmates may be feeling. Separate the two groups at the front so the rest of the class can easily see their faces and know which are in which group. Move as far from the demonstration subjects as is possible and tell them you are going to remove some objects from the bag (or box) you have brought to class and hold them up for the students to see. Ask them to note how they feel when viewing each object.

First, produce a large colorful picture of a snake and slowly move toward them until you are within a few feet of each student. Return to the container and remove a rubber snake and repeat the procedure. Finally, tell them you are going to bring out a live snake and carefully reach inside. It is *not* essential to have a real snake. Some students will begin to respond fearfully from suggestion alone. Stop the demonstration at that point and ask the observing students first to share their observations of the two groups' behavior during the demonstration, especially as objects closer to the real thing were introduced and as all objects were brought closer. Then ask the demonstration subjects to share what they experienced. Student observations are likely to be highly related to subjective reports, allowing the point to be made that behavior alone, if noted carefully, can reveal much that is important about experience.

3. Ask students to imagine they just found out that they did poorly on an important exam for a job or for admission to a professional training program following graduation. Ask them to write on a piece of paper the first reason that occurs to them to explain *why* they did poorly. Stress that their answers are for their own use and will not be handed in. Then ask them to answer the following questions using a 1–7 rating scale.

    a. What is the first reason that occurs to you that explains *why* you did poorly?

    b. Is the cause of your poor performance due to something about you

or something about other people or circumstances? 1 = totally due to other people or circumstances; 7 = totally due to me)
  c. In the future, when looking for a job or applying to school again, will this cause be present? (1 = will never be present again; 7 = will always be present)
  d. Is the cause something that just influences getting a job or admitted to school or does it also influence other areas of your life? (1 = influences just this particular situation; 7 = influences all situations in my life)

After reading out the questions (it only takes a bit longer to read aloud than to have students read copies prepared beforehand), tell students question b assesses the extent they may blame failures on *internal* versus *external* causes, question c the extent of *stable* versus *unstable* attributions, and question d the degree of *global* versus *specific* expectations. Tell them a much longer version of this scale has been used in studies of attributional style in depressed college students. (The study is referenced in the supplemental readings for this chapter.)

Ask students how typical they think the ratings they gave on this demonstration are of how they construe failure in general. The ensuing discussion can be used to illustrate the independence of these three dimensions. Instructors may also wish to demonstrate this empirically by constructing frequency distributions of individual students' scores on the three dimensions. This can be done by having students turn in unsigned slips of paper with their causes and three scores written on them. Correlation coefficients can be calculated and reported on at the beginning of the next class. Regardless of how data are treated, use discussion afterward to illustrate how variation on these independent dimensions can be associated with various mood and behavioral symptoms. Stress that this is a highly shortened version of a research scale and not one that students can use to diagnose themselves or their problems.

Supplemental Readings

Ellis, A. (1973, July). The no-cop-out therapy. *Psychology Today*, 56–62. Albert Ellis points out how irrational beliefs are pervasive in our society, and he summarizes how rational-emotive psychotherapy helps people identify, question, and change their implicit beliefs.

Hall, M. H. (1967, September). An interview with Mr. Behaviorist, B. F. Skinner. *Psychology Today*, 21–23. In this engaging interview, B. F. Skinner is his usual provocative self as he shares his ideas on a number of subjects: his personal life, behavioral techniques as applied to animals, children, and adults, and the future of behaviorism.

Mahoney, M. J. (1977). Reflections on the cognitive-learning trend in psychotherapy. *American Psychologist, 32,* 5–13. Mahoney traces the history and growing popularity of cognitive processes in psychology, especially in the integration of cognitive and behavioral approaches to psychotherapy.

Redd, W. H., & Andrykowski, M. A. (1982). Behavioral intervention in cancer treatment: Controlling aversion to chemotherapy. *Journal of Consulting and Clinical Psychology, 50,* 1018–1029. The application of a number of relaxation-oriented behavioral interventions to cancer patients' aversive reactions to chemotherapy are described. Approximately 25 percent of those undergoing protracted chemotherapy develop nausea or vomiting, symptoms that result from respondent conditioning and can be effectively treated using behavioral methods.

Redd, W. H., & Sleator, W. (1976). Behavior modification used against people. In W. H. Redd & W. Sleator. *Take charge: A personal guide to behavior modification* (pp. 138–159). New York: Random House. This chapter surveys notable abuses of behavioral treatment principles against institutionalized mental patients and prison inmates, persons having little power to resist. The examples presented in this highly readable work are at times horrifying and should be balanced by pointing out that most of these practices have now been eliminated by court action and pressure from the professional community. Stress these abuses as aberrations of behavior therapy and indicate that behavioral programs can be applied in humane ways that still effectively control and improve extremely troubling behaviors.

Seligman, M. E. P., Abramson, L. Y., Semmel, A., & von Baeyer, C. (1979). Depressive attributional style. *Journal of Abnormal Psychology, 88,* 242–247. A research study is described in which depressed and nondepressed college students were compared on the extent to which they made internal versus external, stable versus unstable, and global versus specific attributions about successes and failures. Consistent with the reformulated helplessness model of depression, depressed students were found to more often attribute failures to internal, stable, and global causes and to attribute successes to external and unstable causes. The measure of attributional style use in this study is the basis of the abbreviated scale used in the demonstration described above.

Films

Harry: Behavioral treatment of self-abuse (38 minutes, Research Press, Box 3177R, Champaign, IL 61820). This film portrays Richard Fox's intensive behavioral treatment of a very large institutionalized man displaying various forms of bizarre behavior, including hitting himself in the face. When the film begins, students will be shocked, even frightened, as they view Harry's self-abusive behavior. They are also likely to think the therapist cruel when Harry's restraints are removed as a form of punishment. Fox carefully explains how Harry's behaviors are viewed within the behavioral context and why different procedures are tried. As the film progresses, students will see Harry's behavior become much more appropriate, and he will gradually emerge in their eyes as a person much like themselves. Without doubt, they will be impressed by the dramatic improvement that can be achieved with contingent reinforcement in *one* day over a number of trials. The affection between Harry and Dr. Fox is evident, and students are unlikely to come away seeing behavior techniques as the methods of cruel and sadistic persons. This film is a definite "winner."

Three approaches to psychotherapy, no. 3—Dr. Albert Ellis (42 minutes, Psychological Films, Inc., 110 N. Wheeler St., Orange, CA 92669). Albert Ellis demonstrates his cognitive form of psychotherapy in this classic comparison of Rogers, Perls, and Ellis. All three men interview the same woman, Gloria, and speak briefly about what they were trying to do afterward; each interview is a separate film. The Ellis film nicely illustrates a forerunner of cognitive therapy.

Examination Items

IDENTIFICATION AND SHORT-ANSWER QUESTIONS

1. Define "extinction."
2. Define "systematic desensitization."
3. Define "flooding."
4. What is "partial or intermittent reinforcement"?
5. Differentiate stimulus generalization and discrimination.
6. What does it mean to say "the cognitive psychologist . . . believes that mental events are not mere epiphenomena . . ."?
7. Differentiate "outcome" and "efficacy" expectations.
8. Define cognitive "appraisals."
9. Differentiate "internal" and "external" attributions.
10. Differentiate "stable" and "unstable" attributions.
11. Differentiate "global" and "specific" attributions.
12. Explain Lazarus's multi-model therapy.

ESSAY QUESTIONS

1. What assumptions does the behavioral model make about abnormal behavior?
2. Show how the symptoms of school phobia can be understood using classical and operant conditioning principles.
3. Discuss the implicit irrational beliefs Albert Ellis argues are at the root of neurotic behavior.
4. Discuss the virtues and limitations of the cognitive model.

CHAPTER 6

Investigating Abnormality

Overview

Novices in any field find the methodological distinctions that are of concern to established authorities less attractive than the phenomena under study. Similarly, although the concepts in this chapter are of critical importance to researchers, they are of initially low interest to students. Instructors can overcome this prejudice by emphasizing to students that they must be able to understand research methods well to be able to evaluate the numerous research studies and therapeutic interventions that will be presented throughout the rest of the course. Because presentations of research methods can easily seem unduly abstract and boring, it is especially important to illustrate them and ask students to think like researchers, to draw inferences from data, and to critique others' conclusions. The text gives several examples that can be used in this way, and an additional illustration is given in the demonstrations section for this chapter.

When this topic has been covered, students should have a thorough understanding of the comparisons of strengths and weaknesses presented in Table 6-2 in the text. It is especially important that they should see that *each* of the three methods adds something unique to increasing our understanding of psychopathology and that each should be used in tandem with the others. Avoid encouraging the tendency to see any one method, such as the clinical case study or the laboratory experiment, as "correct" and the others as "false." The previous discussion of models should help students see research methods in this way.

Sample Lecture Outline

Although a number of specific concepts are presented in this chapter, students are more likely to learn them well and to see their relevance if asked to apply them to specific examples. Thus, the sample lecture outline that follows emphasizes discussion and an atmosphere where the instructor frequently plays devil's advocate.

1. Begin by describing a case study and asking, "What are we to conclude about psychopathology from this story?" (The case of hysterical blindness in the book will work nicely or another can be selected from the case books described in the introduction to this manual.) As students propose various conclusions, accept but gently question their contributions, saying, "O.K., that's a good possibility, but are there problems with that conclusion that we should consider?" In drawing this discussion of the clinical case history method to a close, mention that tragic "experiments in nature" are larger scale versions of the same approach. Also point out that clinical observations of unusual cases can be the *first* step in advancing knowledge, but that controlled studies are required to test and expand initial hunches so as to know which to keep and which to discard.

2. Students should have some knowledge of the experiment from previous coursework. Still, spend a few minutes reviewing fundamental experimental concepts, such as "dependent" and "independent variables," "operational definitions," "experimental effects," "control groups," and "random assignment." The text uses a brief research report to review some of these concepts, and instructors can focus on that study (or almost any other study from the research literature). Be certain that students understand that although the experiment is our most powerful way of identifying cause-and-effect relationships, safeguards (double-blind conditions, for example) must be used to control for misinterpretations of results. This is a good time to briefly describe the use of laboratory experiments as highly controlled analogues to guide research with real patients and in clinical settings.

3. Students will also need to review the ways numbers are used to make inferences about psychopathology or treatment methods in the research they will be reviewing in the course. In reviewing the statistical concepts ("frequency distributions," "means," "correlation coefficients," "statistical significance," "misses," and "false alarms") stress the *logic* of their use rather than the computation. A demonstration set of data is included in the following section, which can be used to illustrate the basic concepts.

4. End with a discussion of the correlational approaches that, unlike the experiment, do *not* try to create the phenomena of interest but rather to study the characteristics people bring with them to clinical and research situations. To help make this point, you might discuss Cronbach's 1957 article on psychologists preferring experimental and correlational methods, which is listed under the supplemental readings. Bring this meeting to a close by previewing the next topic to be covered, assessment and diagnosis, pointing out how the general topics discussed today have strong practical implications for the ways psychologists categorize psychopathology in practice and research settings.

Demonstrations

1. *Mixed Design Experiment.* The following hypothetical data set has been created to give students "hands on" experience with data and experimental logic. The major objective of this exercise is to show students how researchers must make general conclusions from groups of individual data points and how studies can mix correlational methods (studying groups showing different symptoms) with experimental manipulations (randomly dividing diagnostic groups into parts and treating them differently). This demonstration can be completed in twenty to thirty minutes of class time or assigned to students to complete on their own. Either way, duplicate the data presented here and distribute copies to the students. Introduce this exercise as follows:

> This is a fictional study of the effect of different contingencies on weight loss in students reporting depression and eating disorders. The study combines correlational and experimental methods. The numbers that follow measure the weight loss of several groups of female college students over a six-week period. Data from sixty persons are listed by group and the numbers are expressed in terms of percentage of body weight lost (minus numbers) or gained (positive numbers). The women were recruited from three different sources: (1) "normal" college students responding to an advertisement in the college newspaper for women wishing to lose weight, (2) patients being seen at the psychological clinic for depressive symptoms who were told the program might improve their self-image and self-esteem, and (3) patients being seen at the clinic for problems with uncontrolled eating. All subjects expressed a desire to lose weight and agreed to try the experimental procedures to help them with this. As can be seen, two control groups are included to serve as contrasts for the group of women with eating disorders: a nontreatment group and a group in treatment for a different problem.
>
> Each of the three groups was divided into thirds and exposed to one of three experimental conditions: (1) subjects were offered $50 if they could drop their body weight by at least 10 percent at the end of the six weeks; they were asked to keep a daily log of everything they ate; a "weight counselor" came by every three days to weigh them, look over their eating records, and tell them what they were doing wrong (criticism condition); (2) subjects in this condition were treated just as the women in the first condition except that the counselor praised them or what they did right (praise condition); and (3) students in the control condition were only offered the money and encouraged to keep the eating log; they had no contact with the program until they reported in to be weighed at the end of six weeks.

Experimental Conditions	"Normal" Volunteers			Depressive Volunteers			Uncontrolled Eating Volunteers		
Money + Criticism	−9	−7	−10	−7	−10	+2	−15	−5	+4
	−14	−9	−7	+7	+9	−6	+13	+16	+9
	+1	−10	−9	+3	−2	0	−4	0	−4
	−6	+4	−8	−8	−14	0	+7	+12	+7
	−8	−7	−6	−4	+9	−9	0	+7	+9
Money + Praise	−10	−9	−11	+1	+2	+3	−10	0	−9
	−8	−15	−13	−9	0	−11	+1	−14	−8
	−11	−12	−9	+1	−13	−9	−12	−1	−11
	−9	−5	+5	−3	+4	+2	0	−4	+1
	−9	+7	−11	12	−1	−15	−11	−14	−13
Money Alone	−18	−15	−10	−3	+5	+1	+8	−2	−6
	−12	−8	+1	−1	−3	−2	−3	+1	+2
	+3	−10	−14	0	−2	−3	+1	0	−3
	−11	−9	−11	+1	0	+3	0	−2	+1
	−14	−13	−9	−6	0	−5	+3	+1	0

Ask students to construct frequency distributions for each of the six groups and for each of the three rows and columns. Then ask them to answer the following questions by inspecting their tabulations, ignoring for the moment the question of statistical inference. After each question, ask students why they conclude as they do.

a. Was the $50 an incentive for the women to lose weight?
b. Was the $50 more effective as an incentive for some groups than others? If so, with which groups was it most and least effective?
c. Was adding criticism more effective than the money alone?
d. Was adding praise more effective than money alone and than the addition of criticism?
e. Were the effects of praise and criticism more effective for some groups than others?
f. Which single group had the largest number of people meet the goal of 10 percent reduction?
g. Which single group had the largest number of notable failures (subjects gaining at least five pounds over the study period)? Does looking at "clinical significance" in this way tell us things inspection of means omits?
h. Might we conclude from this study that persons with eating disorders are more responsive (positively or negatively) to environmental contingencies than depressed or normal college students?

After leading this discussion, indicate how statistics could be used to answer the questions with more confidence. Compute means and standard deviations before class and show how they could be used to test differences between groups using analysis-of-variance models.

2. *Single-Subject Demonstration.*   Ask students to pick a behavior they would like to increase (studying, exercise, speaking to strangers, asking men or women for dates, and so forth) and to keep an accurate base-line record of how frequently it occurs for three days. Instruct them to then experiment for two days with rewarding themselves by doing something they find positive on days when they increase their behavior by an amount they specify beforehand. Have them discontinue reinforcing themselves and return to base line for two additional days before discussing their experience in class or in a short written report.

This experience requires considerable student self-discipline but, if encouraged strongly by the instructor and given the opportunity to report what they learned, it can teach them much about single-subject research.

Supplemental Readings

Lee Cronbach. (1957). The two disciplines of scientific psychology. *American Psychologist, 12,* 671–684. This article is still one of the best discussions available of the fundamental differences between experimental and correlational research designs and the psychologists who prefer one over the other. It is much better for use with undergraduates than his more recent article with a similar subject and title (Cronbach, L. [1975]. Beyond the two disciplines of scientific psychology. *American Psychologist, 30,* 116–127). In addition to advocating mixed designs, Cronbach points out that "correlationists" are mostly interested in the individual and group differences that subjects bring with them to research settings, while "experimentalists" are mainly interested in being able to produce the phenomena of interest and to control individual differences error by randomly assigning subjects to treatment conditions.

Examination Items

IDENTIFICATION AND SHORT-ANSWER QUESTIONS

1. Select one or two of the following four limitations to the clinical case method and explain the disadvantages:
   a. selectivity
   b. lack of repeatability
   c. lack of generality
   d. insufficient evidence for causality

2. What is an operational definition?
3. What is an experimental effect?
4. What is "meta-analysis?"
5. Define "confounds."
6. Why is random assignment to treatment groups so important in an experiment?
7. Define "yoking."
8. Define "demand characteristics."
9. What is a frequency distribution?
10. What does it mean to say something is "statistically significant"?
11. Differentiate "false alarms" and "misses."
12. Differentiate "positive" and "negative" correlation.

ESSAY QUESTIONS
1. What are the strengths and weaknesses of the clinical case method?
2. What is a "double-blind" experiment and why is it so essential in clinical research?
3. How can an experimental effect be demonstrated using a single subject?
4. What are advantages and disadvantages of "experiments of nature"?
5. What are advantages and disadvantages of "laboratory models"?
6. (Alternative to #5) Discuss the advantages and disadvantages of learned helplessness as a laboratory model of depression.

CHAPTER 7

Psychological Assessment and Classification

Overview

Assessment and diagnosis are topics of high interest to students, in part because they have taken standardized achievement and aptitude tests and want to know more about them. Students are also especially curious about assessment and diagnosis because they engage in similar processes with friends, especially new persons they meet. Like most people, students use implicit theories of personality and personality assessment in everyday relationships. Their desire to "figure out what makes people tick" makes them quite open to learning about the complexities of assessment and diagnosis, especially if given a chance to apply what they are learning to live examples.

A major objective of this chapter is to sensitize students to the presence of large individual differences in personality and behavior and the necessity for researchers and practicing clinicians to reduce their observations of others to dimensions or categories of workable size. Both of the two topics covered in this chapter—psychological assessment and diagnosis—can be used to make this general point.

Sample Lecture Outline

Students will be more excited about the specific concepts in this chapter if asked to apply them to a concrete example—to understand a living person. The most ambitious way to achieve these objectives is to assign the *Super-Shrink* computer-simulated interview as described in the opening section of this Instructor's Manual. *SuperShrink* provides a comprehensive and complex individual for students to interview and understand, making it possible for them to grapple with assessment and diagnostic issues far beyond what is usually possible for undergraduates to do. Discussing the *SuperShrink* laboratory assignment at the same time as the general issues regarding assessment and classification will heighten students' involvement and interest in this material.

45

The lecture outline that follows provides another example of the concepts by giving a demonstration with a concrete example — conducting a short interview and testing session with a confederate. The same objective could also be achieved by showing parts of a videotaped assessment session or asking students to *imagine* what they would say if asked to interview someone.

1. Begin today's class by announcing a visitor will be arriving in a few minutes and that the class's goal is to learn as much about the person as possible in a few minutes. Tell them you (or another confederate who comes in with the interviewee) will be asking the person questions for the purpose of getting an overall picture of "what makes the person tick." Ask the class to take notes on what occurs to them as they listen to the interview and to watch the client's behavior closely. Then conduct a ten- to fifteen-minute interview with someone playing a college student troubled by test anxiety, social withdrawal, or some other mild form of psychopathology familiar to students. Bring the interview to a close and ask the confederate(s) to leave. Then ask, "What did you observe or learn about our visitor?"

2. After students have shared their observations and hypotheses about the individual under study, shift the focus to the *process* of learning about a person using the clinical interview. This class discussion makes an excellent foundation for differentiating structured from clinical interviews, the concepts of reliability and validity, and the major varieties of psychological assessment.

3. Students will be highly interested in a fuller discussion and demonstration of psychological assessment, although the rest of the class should be spent on diagnosis if only one class session is to be devoted to this chapter. If two sessions are to be used, formal testing can be demonstrated by bringing in a single Rorschach card, one or two TAT cards, and selected MMPI items and profiles. In your lecture on how a comprehensive battery of tests is given in clinical practice, emphasize that it requires extensive training to give and interpret psychological tests appropriately.

4. When introducing the topic of diagnosis, point out that students will be using it throughout the remainder of the course as specific diagnostic categories are covered. Ask, "Why do we need to have a diagnostic system?" Students will come up with most of the reasons given in the text (a communication shorthand, a guide for etiology and treatment, and an aid to scientific research) and may add others of their own. Bring this discussion to a close by emphasizing that although the process of diagnosis has faults and potential dangers, some agreed-upon system for compressing varying observations into categories is necessary in both clinical and research settings.

5. DSM-III-R should be the subject of the rest of today's session. Give an overview of the categories and point out that the next segment of the course covers what is known about many of the various disorders included. Stress the biomedical model and the *individual* dysfunction assumptions of the DSM

system. Also stress the improvements of the DSM-III and DSM-III-R over the DSM-II system, especially how the current system was an attempt to overcome demonstrated weaknesses in previous approaches and reflects a theoretical shift away from psychodynamic assumptions of causality to a more behavioral and cause-neutral perspective. Do stress the recent study showing that the reliability of DSM-III is much improved over DSM-II, though still below acceptable research standards. You may also want to say a few words about the factors that bias diagnosis. Students will want to respond to the classic Rosenhan experiment on pseudopatients and may need reassurance that just because expectancy effects and bias *can* exist does not mean the whole system of assessment and diagnosis is bankrupt.

Demonstrations

1. Behavioral assessment can be demonstrated using the single-subject observations listed in Chapter 6. Students should attempt a *functional analysis* of the behavior they recorded and attempted to change. Encourage them to look for stimuli (people, settings, critical events, time of day) surrounding the behavior in question.

2. Offer students an optional experience in psychological assessment in which you (or assistants) administer individuals an abbreviated version—a thirty-minute session is sufficient for the purpose of this experience—of a common psychological test and answer any questions they have about the procedure. Allow students to select whether they will receive part of the Rorschach, TAT, MMPI, or the WISC-R—giving the children's version is less threatening and keeps them from having contact with the adult version. Stress that no *one* test tells very much about an individual and that you will not be able to give any feedback whatsoever about their performance. Offering this experience does take time. Usually no more than 30 to 50 percent of a class will volunteer for this experience. If too many request it, tell them you will randomly select twenty students from the list of those interested, and ask some of them to report back to the class afterward on what they learned from the experience. Although those students choosing this experience receive no formal credit, they will learn a great deal and everyone will appreciate the instructor's willingness to offer it.

Supplemental Readings

Mischel, W. (1977). On the future of personality measurement. *American Psychologist, 32,* 246–254. Mischel discusses a number of closely related issues in personality measurement: multiple determinants, context, various goals of different researchers and clinicians, and person variables—influences resulting from individual differences. Mischel shows how current views on these traditional issues show the emergence of a new image of human nature.

Schacht, T., & Nathan, P. (1977). But is it good for psychologists? Appraisal and status of DSM-III. *American Psychologist*, 32, 1017–1026. This article appeared just before DSM-III was published and gives an overview of the changes included. It is a good critical overview of the new system and asks important questions about its validity and utility which are still being investigated empirically.

Examination Items

IDENTIFICATION AND SHORT-ANSWER QUESTIONS

1. Differentiate "inter-judge" and "test-retest" reliability.
2. Differentiate "clinical" and "structured interviews."
3. What does the Minnesota Multiphasic Personality Inventory (MMPI) measure?
4. What is the Q-sort?
5. What are the assumptions of the Role Construct Repertory Test?
6. What are projective tests?
7. Describe the Rorschach Test and how it is used.
8. What does the Thematic Apperception Test (TAT) assess?
9. What are the scales on the Wechler intelligence tests?
10. Define "functional analysis."
11. What criteria does DSM-III-R use to define a mental disorder?
12. Differentiate descriptive and predictive validity.

ESSAY QUESTIONS

1. Discuss the reasons we need a standard diagnostic system.
2. What are the major differences between DSM-II, DSM-III, and DSM-III-R? Why are they important?
3. What are some of the conditions that have been shown to bias psychiatric diagnoses?

CHAPTER 8

Fear and Phobia: Anxiety Felt

Overview

This chapter marks a major transition in the text and the course. Everything thus far has been preliminary to the chapters and class sessions dealing with specific clusters of disorders. Because so much needs to be covered in the rest of the course, the pace of things will of necessity slow down a bit, and most chapters from here on will require at least two class sessions.

The disorders discussed in this chapter are attempts by the patient to deal with anxiety, the fundamental symptom of most forms of psychopathology. Although the disorders in which anxiety is observed occur commonly, research in recent years shows they can be treated. For example, the phobias have been shown to result from learning and are amenable to appropriate psychotherapeutic intervention based on classical and instrumental conditioning techniques. Yet, there is recent evidence that biological predispositions influence the types of objects—prepared versus unprepared—that are most likely to become feared and the individuals likely to develop panic attacks or phobias from exposure.

The disorders in this chapter lend themselves well to comparisons between psychodynamic and cognitive-behavioral models. Because this is the first disorder considered in detail, some time should be set aside for this comparison. The sample outline presented for this chapter assumes that two class sessions are devoted to these disorders. The first can deal with the issues of fear and anxiety and the phobias, and the second with the post-traumatic stress disorder.

Introduce students to the specific topics associated with these disorders in which anxiety is observed. In addition, help students see how the learning model is applied in actuality and how it differs from the psychodynamic model's view of the same disorders.

Sample Lecture Outline

There is a great deal that could be covered in this chapter and instructors will have to omit some interesting and important topics. The outline that follows assumes that at least two class sessions will be devoted to this topic. Even then, instructors will have to move quickly to complete the suggested outline. A good place to break the outline is just before the discussion of specific phobias.

1. Begin by emphasizing the transition to diagnostic categories.

2. To increase student involvement, ask them to imagine in as much detail as possible the most anxious moment they have ever had or seen in another. Give them a minute or so to think about this before asking them to keep these experiences in mind as the topics in this chapter are covered. Ask them to share their observations with one another if discussion is desired.

3. Introduce the anxiety disorders by differentiating the *manifest anxiety* disorders to be considered first from the *anxiety inferred* categories coming up in Chapter 9. By way of introduction, mention that a tremendous breakthrough has occurred in the past twenty years in how well we understand and are able to effectively treat the manifest anxiety disorders. Although improvement in the manifest anxiety disorders may not be as dramatic as it was for general paresis, it is still a modern success story.

4. The rest of this class (and part of the next) will be spent on fear and phobias. First, discuss the various elements of fear. Table 8-1 in the text presents the elements clearly and is useful to focus on. Ask, "How do your observations of extreme anxiety fit this scheme?" Stress the adaptive nature of our biological fear response system and point out that the manifest anxiety disorders represent extreme examples of how our emotional responses can become dysfunctional through conditioning.

5. Focus on Table 8-3 on the common phobias, pointing out onset and sex differences as well as the relative incidence figures. Ask, "Why might these sex differences exist?" Students will point to a number of possible causes, including biological differences in emotionality and social differences in sex role conditioning and the likelihood of physical assault. Then be sure students understand the classic psychoanalytic formulation of phobias (avoid getting bogged down in the details of the Little Hans case) and the conditioned emotional response of the behavioral model. Table 8-4 is particularly important. Help students understand how the various elements of the classical conditioning paradigm are applied to specific phobias by presenting the examples below and asking them to note which element is the CS, US, UR, and CR.

    a. A female college student is frightened one night by a strange man she believes followed her to her dormitory from the library. In subsequent weeks, she becomes increasingly reluctant to go to the library and eventually ceases going out of her dormitory at all in the evenings. When first seen at the psychology clinic, her phobia was so severe she refused to attend concerts or go out on dates after dark.

b. A twenty-eight-year-old biochemist works with toxins on a cancer research project. Although he reports no fear of these toxins, he comes to the mental health center complaining of a strong fear of botulism which is so severe he will not eat anything prepared by anyone else. At first, he would not eat in restaurants or in other people's homes. By the time he appeared for treatment, he would not eat his wife's cooking either. He has no memory of traumatic events associated with food or toxins, but he knows his phobia started six months ago when he first went to work on the cancer project.

c. A forty-five-year-old furniture store manager wins a trip to the Virgin Islands as a reward for an excellent sales year. She has never flown before and is terrified of the airplane flight. She is afraid she will have a panic attack in front of the other passengers and will not be able to get out of the plane. The fear of crashing does not concern her very much. Being embarrassed in front of the other store managers from across the country is foremost among her worries.

6. Point out how avoidance conditioning is required to explain why conditioned fear responses do not extinguish but become persistent phobias. Ask students to speculate on how escape or avoidance of anxiety can be providing reinforcement in the examples presented previously.

7. Describe the three behavioral therapies for phobias and ask students how each would be applied to the examples in the text or in this section of the manual. Instructors can choose to present these therapies themselves if desired or necessary because of time limitations. A demonstration is suggested in the next section that asks students to construct a stimulus hierarchy.

8. Discuss the criticisms of the behavioral model of phobias. Then focus on the research supporting the concept of "prepared classical conditioning" as an explanation of why phobias become conditioned to a relatively limited number of stimulus objects.

9. Focus on the recent evidence for biological differences between individuals likely to experience panic or anxiety attacks as a result of exposure to fearful circumstances. Discuss the continuing debate between those favoring biological and cognitive explanations of these findings.

10. Stress the major symptoms of post-traumatic stress disorder (emotional numbness, reliving of the experience, and anxiety) and ask if students have ever known anyone who showed them. Students may want to share their experiences or observations of others with the class. Whether students' examples or those presented in the text are used, spend a few minutes showing how natural disasters and manmade stress (especially combat) may stim-

ulate symptoms of manifest and persistent anxiety. Students will be especially interested in the supplemental readings on Vietnam veterans, which expands on examples included in the text.

11. Although the previous two (or three) classes will have been rushed, take a few minutes to reflect on all that has been covered to give students a chance to ask questions and integrate the various ideas. Help them gain a perspective on human nature, which includes the biological advantages of anxiety and fear alongside an understanding of how these emotional reactions can become too easily conditioned and persistent in some people.

Demonstrations

1. Ask students to pick an object, animal, or situation that they are afraid of and to construct a stimulus hierarchy containing 8 to 10 points. Let 1 be the instance of the feared situation arousing the least discomfort, and 10 the instance creating the greatest discomfort. Encourage them to use their imagination to decide where various elements fall in the hierarchy. Instructors can ask students to discuss these hierarchies in class, but because class time is very limited on this chapter, another option is to ask students to turn in their hierarchies for "pass/fail" grading.

2. Have students complete the Anxiety State Questionnaire presented in the text on two different occasions: when they are very calm and relaxed, and again when they are more anxious than usual (just before an exam, artistic performance, athletic event, "big date," or job interview). Have them discuss in class or write a brief paper outlining how their scores when anxious varied across the situations.

Supplemental Readings

Lipkin, J. O., Blank, A. S., Parson, E. R., & Smith, J. (1982). Vietnam veterans and post-traumatic stress disorder. *Hospital and Community Psychiatry, 33,* 908–912. The authors, one of whom is a psychologist who is a Vietnam vet, argue that Vietnam veterans are especially at risk for developing post-traumatic stress disorder. They discuss their explanation of this increased risk as they explore four broad types of disorders commonly found among this population.

Smith, J. (1982). Personality responsibility in traumatic stress reactions. *Psychiatric Annals, 12,* 1021–1030. A number of short case examples from civil catastrophes as well as combat are presented to illustrate the guilt commonly felt by survivors of stressful events, especially when others die. This is a highly readable article that undergraduates will find very interesting.

Films

Phobias (17 minutes, Time-Life Multi-Media, 100 Eisenhower Drive, Paramus, NJ 07652). This film presents several typical phobic reactions. Two psychiatrists discuss these illustrative examples.

Examination Items

IDENTIFICATION AND SHORT-ANSWER QUESTIONS
1. Define "phobic disorder."
2. Define "post-traumatic stress disorder."
3. Define "panic disorder."
4. Define "generalized anxiety disorder."
5. What are the cognitive elements of fear?
6. What are the somatic elements of fear?
7. What are the behavioral elements of fear?
8. Differentiate "fear" and "anxiety."
9. Differentiate "incidence" and "prevalence."
10. Differentiate "agoraphobia" and "social phobia."
11. Differentiate "nosophobia" and "hypochondriasis."
12. Who was Little Hans and why is he important?
13. Explain the therapy of systematic desensitization.
14. What is a stimulus hierarchy?
15. Explain flooding therapy.
16. What is prepared classical conditioning?
17. What evidence suggests panic attacks have some biological origin?
18. What are the major symptoms of post-traumatic stress disorder?
19. What is the rape trauma syndrome?

ESSAY QUESTIONS
1. (Note: Do not use this essay if IDs 5–7 are used) What are the various elements that make up the human fear response?
2. A five-year-old boy becomes distraught on the first day of school when left at his classroom by his mother. Thereafter, he refuses to go to school, fights and kicks if taken there, and occasionally vomits in the car or at the door to his classroom. Over the first three months of school, the child is so phobic that he does not spend more than thirty minutes at one time in his classroom. How can this instance of "school phobia" be conceptualized using *classical* and *avoidance* conditioning concepts?
3. What are the major limitations of the behavioral account of phobias?
4. What is the cognitive account of some individuals' greater likelihood of developing panic attacks?

Obsession, Hysteria, and Dissociation: Anxiety Inferred

Overview

Students will find the disorders studied in Chapter 9 of special interest. Most will have some obsessive traits themselves or friends who show troubling obsessions or compulsions. Many will have enough lingering identity problems to be enamored with the idea that some people can have more than one distinct personality. Instructors can count on students to read Chapter 9 carefully on their own with little encouragement.

This chapter deals with the most traditional of the anxiety related disorders and complements the coverage of the anxiety disorders in the previous chapter. What is most important for students to grasp here is that obsessive and hysterical symptoms are thought by many — especially psychodynamic clinicians — to serve to defend patients against underlying anxiety, even though persons troubled by these disorders show no overt anxiety. It is also important to stress that, while the phobias provide considerable support for the behavioral model, it is these traditional anxiety related disorders — the ones first studied by Freud — that provide the most support for psychodynamic ideas.

Sample Lecture Outline

Although Chapter 9 *can* be completed in one class, instructors who move through the obsessive and disassociative disorders more leisurely will find the time well spent. The following outline assumes only a single class meeting will be used for these disorders.

1. Begin by stressing that the subject of today's class consists of those patterns of human behavior first studied by Freud in repressive Victorian Europe and thought to reflect anxiety about unconscious fears and desires. Be sure students understand the distinction between the manifest and inferred anxiety disorders covered in Chapters 8 and 9. Point out that the symptoms of the

disorders covered in Chapter 9 are thought to reflect *defenses* against under-lying anxiety, the presence of which frequently must be inferred.

2. Open the discussion of obsessive-compulsive disorders by saying that most people have recurring thoughts or ritualistic behaviors and asking students to describe some that they have seen in themselves and others. (If you volunteer some of your own, students will be more comfortable sharing theirs.) After a few minutes of discussing the common thoughts and behaviors students propose, show how they are different from much more worrisome obsessions and compulsions (unwelcome intrusions from within that are difficult to control). Most students have at some point ruminated about something of concern to them and can be encouraged to remember these times when imagining what obsessions are like. Similarly, when discussing compulsions, they can be reminded of their own superstitious behaviors. Stress that persons troubled by such thoughts or behaviors *do* become anxious if not allowed to perform them.

3. Ask students to think about what factors can lead to obsessions and compulsions as a prelude to considering the cognitive-behavioral and psychoanalytic theories. Stress that the two views are not mutually exclusive but complementary, not only to each other but to biological theories, which stress biological vulnerability to obsessive-compulsive symptoms. Discuss treatment in conjunction with etiology to illustrate how both the psychodynamic and behavioral treatments follow from the causative assumptions made. Point out that behavioral treatments focus primarily on compulsions, not obsessions. Bring the discussion of obsessive-compulsive disorders to a close by reviewing the clues that indicate that anxiety does underlie the overt symptoms.

4. Focus on the problems diagnosing somatoform disorders, differentiating malingering, psychosomatic and factitious disorders, and undiagnosed physical illness. Table 9-2 is useful for clarifying the differences between these disorders and, by contrast, the essential characteristics of somatoform problems. Be sure to emphasize that conversion symptoms have changed over time and vary among individuals as a function of education and psychological sophistication.

5. Lastly, consider the dissociative disorders. Students will be fascinated by these disorders and eager to hear additional case studies. The text mentions several, including the Hillside Strangler's recent attempt to fake multiple personality. Instructors can find other examples in the full-length works and case books referenced in the introduction to this manual. Stress how rare the dissociative disorders are and that all share a distortion and isolation of consciousness similar to what is seen in hypnotic phenomena.

6. If time is available, spend five minutes or so tying together the disorders in which anxiety is observed and those in which it is inferred. Point out that these disorders have been a battlefield over which the psychodynamic and

behavioral models have fought and that it is with the anxiety disorders that the behavioral approach has been the most successful. Similarly, the psychodynamic approach finds the most theoretical support in conversion and dissociative disorders. The organization of Chapters 8 and 9 reflects the front-line positions in this continuing struggle between these major paradigms.

Demonstrations

Have students imagine they are split into different personalities. If done in class, have them close their eyes and fantasize for a couple of minutes. If used as an out-of-class exercise, suggest they go to a quiet place and close their eyes for a few minutes of fantasy. Either way, encourage them to imagine that more than one person occupies their self and to imagine what the different people are like. Suggest they have conversations with the different parts of themselves, out loud if feasible. Afterwards, ask students to share their experiences and how successful they were at splitting their conscious sense of self. Some students will do amazingly well at this and be able to report interesting conversations with their alter egos.

Supplemental Readings

Freud, S. (1963). The problem of anxiety. Dora: An analysis of a case of hysteria. In J. Breuer & S. Freud, *Studies on hysteria*. New York: Macmillan. This paperback edition nicely illustrates Freud's ideas on hysteria and his writing style.

Pollack, J. M. (1979). Obsessive-compulsive personality: A review. *Psychological Bulletin, 86,* 225–241. This article reviews twenty years of research on obsessive-compulsive personality (or anal character) and concludes that the evidence largely supports psychodynamic theory and clinical descriptions. Evidence is still lacking about the origins of this common characterological pattern, but it does hold together well in published studies.

Films

Case study of a multiple personality (30 minutes, Pennsylvania State University, Audio-Visual Services, 6 Willard Building, University Park, PA 16802). This film presents dramatized interviews with the three personalities of "Eve" and an interview with Chris Sizemore, the "real" Eve of Thigpen and Cleckley's classic case study.

Obsessive-compulsive neurosis (28 minutes, McGraw-Hill Films, P.O. Box 641, Del Mar, CA 92014). This film presents an illustrative case study of a middle-aged man troubled by obsessive-compulsive symptoms.

Examination Items

IDENTIFICATION AND SHORT-ANSWER QUESTIONS

1. Define "obsessive personality."
2. What are the assumptions of the cognitive-behavioral view of obsessive-compulsive symptoms?
3. What questions about obsessive-compulsive disorders does the cognitive-behavioral view leave unanswered?
4. What are the defining criteria for the somatoform disorders?
5. What is somatization disorder (or Briquet's syndrome)?
6. Define somatoform pain disorder (or psychalgia).
7. What are the differences between malingering and authentic somatoform disorders?
8. Differentiate "malingering" and "secondary gain."
9. What is a factitious disorder?
10. Define "depersonalization."
11. Differentiate global, retrograde, anterograde, and selective amnesia.

ESSAY QUESTIONS

1. What distinguishes obsessions of clinical proportions from more harmless recurring thoughts?
2. Discuss the cognitive-behavioral view of obsessive-compulsive disorder, focusing on the steps thought to lead from harmless obsessions and compulsions to dysfunctional symptoms.
3. What is the evidence that persons showing obsessive-compulsive symptoms may have a biological predisposition for this disorder?
4. What is the psychodynamic view of the origin of obsessive-compulsive symptoms?
5. What clues exist that anxiety underlies the obsessive, somatoform, and dissociative disorders?
6. What other disorders must be seriously considered when making a diagnosis of somatoform disorder? How does a clinician tell the difference?
7. Compare the psychoanalytic and communicative views of the cause of somatoform disorders.
8. What are notable differences between psychogenically and organically caused amnesia?
9. What is the best view available of how multiple personality begins and develops?

CHAPTER 10

Health Psychology and Psychosomatic Disorders

Overview

Most students will have less initial interest in this chapter than in the two on anxiety related disorders because they may fail to appreciate the theoretical importance of the emerging field of health psychology. Guard against this tendency by previewing Chapter 10 with special enthusiasm during preceding meetings. Tell students that health psychology is a very "hot topic," an area in which tremendous change and progress has occurred in the past ten years. Animal research receives a great deal of emphasis in this chapter, and students will find it less of a chore if its theoretical importance is stressed. Also give them the expectancy that the ideas to be covered will be relevant to them personally, to many health problems they and their families show.

Stress how psychosomatic disorders can tell us about the critically important mind-body issue and how cognitive expectations and physiological predispositions interact to produce illness. This chapter is one of the best illustrations of the contribution animal research can make to the study of psychopathology. Because this is the first chapter in which the diathesis-stress model is discussed in detail and applied to a diagnostic category, another objective is to give students a solid grounding they can use when applying it to other diagnostic categories.

The text addresses in detail only a few kinds of specific disorders, particularly ulcers and coronary heart disease. Attention is also given to the new area of psychoneuroimmunology. The sample lecture outline for this chapter focuses on the general principles more than the specific disorders. Another option is to present research on specific disorders other than those treated in the text. The special issue of the *Journal of Consulting and Clinical Psychology* on behavioral medicine (December, 1982) provides comprehensive coverage of this area and can be used to supplement students' knowledge of specific problems. Regardless of the approach taken, more than one class meeting will be required to do justice to this area of growing importance. The sample outline assumes at least two classes will be allocated.

Sample Lecture Outline

1. Begin by stressing that this area is important for theoretical as well as clinical reasons. Mention that health psychology is an area bordering psychology and medicine which is of increasing interest to psychologists and physicians.

2. To increase student involvement, ask for a show of hands on how many students know someone who has one of the following: (1) migraine headaches, (2) asthma, (3) high blood pressure, (4) chronic skin rashes, (5) stomach ulcers, (6) chronic constipation, (7) high cholesterol, or (8) has had a heart attack. Almost everyone in the room will respond, giving students a memorable illustration of the pervasiveness of psychosomatic disorders and the concern about coronary heart disease. Be sure that students understand that psychosomatic disorders are differentiated from somatoform disorders by the presence of physical changes in the body. Put the psychosomatic disorders into evolutionary perspective by asking, "Why might nature select for individuals with tendencies to develop these often life-threatening maladies?" The ensuing discussion can be used to illustrate how the psychosomatic disorders are unfortunate consequences of the physiological mechanisms essential for our species' survival and evolution.

3. Continue these introductory comments by presenting briefly the *diathesis-stress* model. Emphasize that both a biological predisposition — the diathesis — and sufficient stress are required to be present for the disorder to develop. Telling students this model will be used later on in the discussion of schizophrenia and manic-depressive disorder will heighten their motivation to remember it.

4. Of the disorders covered in the text, the wealth of research on coronary heart disease is the most important to emphasize. List on the board the seven risk factors of coronary heart disease, and ask students how many of them can be controlled or changed. Then summarize the major findings about psychological contributions to heart disease, emphasizing how relevant psychological interventions are to this major health problem.

5. Continue the discussion of psychological contributions to coronary heart disease by noting that similar cognitive variables are being shown to affect the immune as well as the circulatory system. Be certain students appreciate the implications of this relationship to cancer and AIDS, other major contemporary health problems.

6. The "biomedical model" is especially powerful when applied to the psychosomatic disorders, so consider it in detail, beginning with evidence supporting a genetic contribution. A table can be presented on the board or screen (or a handout can be prepared) summarizing the genetic evidence from twin studies for various disorders discussed in the text. Point out that establishing a genetic link says little about the mechanism of that influence. This makes a logical transition to the theory of specific organ vulnerability,

to answering the question of why a given individual develops a specific type of psychosomatic problem. Selye's ideas on biological reactions to enduring stress are particularly important. Present his hypothesis about the general adaptation syndrome and show how it gives one plausible interpretation of much that is known about the responses of humans and animals to stress over time.

5. Do not spend much time on the psychodynamic model other than to say that it has received modest support when applied to males but no support when applied to females. A more appropriate question to consider is the extent to which personality factors, especially the Type A personality style, contribute to heart attacks. Students will be quite interested in this topic.

6. Students should be made aware that biological predisposition by itself in no way accounts for psychosomatic disorders. The role of conditioning in these disorders and the modest effects of stress as inferred from life changes should be stressed. The classroom demonstration using the life events rating scale (modified for college students) will help make this point and will be of particular interest to students.

Demonstrations

1. Blood pressure is an important and easily measured physiological sign that can be used to demonstrate several important points. One option is to bring in a blood pressure cuff and gauge and demonstrate how to measure it. This increases student involvement in any discussion of risk factors in hypertension or research in which blood pressure is an outcome measure. Another option is to use a confederate to take the blood pressure of any curious students during the class session. If sufficient equipment and class or laboratory time is available, divide students into pairs and have each learn to take the readings from the other.

A more elaborate option is to make introductory comments about measuring blood pressure and ask for ten volunteers. Have five of the students take readings from the other five and list them on the board. Then, without removing the cuffs, have a confederate suddenly enter the room and begin shouting insults at the instructor. Do not emphasize instructor authority over students, however, by having the confederate voice anger about a poor grade. Privately warn the students taking the blood pressure readings about what is going to happen and instruct them to take another reading immediately after the instructor has succeeded in getting the angry student to leave the room. Display the new readings for comparison. This demonstration illustrates how anxiety can elevate blood pressure temporarily, and it offers students insight into how chronic anxiety could lead to hypertension. Instructors can also demonstrate relaxation training as a treatment for hypertension by following the anxiety demonstration with instruction in progressive relaxation. After everyone has gone through a five- to ten-minute abbreviated version of any of the relaxation procedures, have the target students' blood pressure remeasured and displayed.

2. Illustrate McClelland's research on TAT personality predictors of hypertension by showing them card 1 (boy with violin). Read the sample TAT stories provided below and ask students to guess which would indicate high needs for affiliation, achievement, power. Ask if the needs are expressed or inhibited in each story.

   a. This boy wanted to go outside and play ball with his friends, but his parents told him he had to practice his violin. He just sits there daydreaming about running for a touchdown pass with his buddies (expressed affiliative need).
   b. For as long as this boy can remember, he has wanted to be a famous violinist, to play with the world's greatest symphonies and conductors. He's getting ready to practice and is enjoying thinking about the applause he will hear some day, about how good he is going to be (expressed achievement need).
   c. This boy doesn't want to be practicing. He'd rather be playing with his friends, but he knows this is not in his best long-term interests, that he'll never amount to anything if he doesn't learn how to commit himself to a goal and stick to it. He knows it is important not to let his desire for friends get in his way (inhibited affiliative need).
   d. This boy is thinking about how he is going to win the audition at school tomorrow. He does not want to be first chair violinist in the school orchestra just to beat the boy and girl now sitting ahead of him. He wants it so he will not feel like a "nothing," like someone who cannot excel, cannot make it to the top (inhibited power need).
   e. This boy has been practicing hard all afternoon. His friends are out playing, but he is inside working away. He's determined to be the best, to beat everyone who shows up for the orchestra auditions tomorrow. He's just got to make first chair . . . be number 1! . . . and he knows he will make it (expressed power need).
   f. This boy is worrying about his violin playing. He knows his parents, grandparents, and teachers expect him to become a great violinist, but he's afraid that no matter how hard he practices he still won't make it. He can't let himself fail (inhibited achievement need).

After giving and explaining the correct classification of the themes in these stories, refer to the research mentioned in the text showing that men who revealed greater needs for power than affiliation and whose power needs were inhibited were more likely to be hypertensive twenty years later.

3. Ask students to rate themselves on the Social Readjustment Rating Scale presented in the text using the past six months as a reference period. Also ask students to use a ten-point scale to estimate how frequently they have

been sick with colds, sore throats, flu, etc., during the same six months. Collect their scores on the two scales and construct a scatterplot. Compute a correlation coefficient for presentation during the next class. In connection with this demonstration, mention that Holmes and Rahe's scale has been widely criticized for treating positive and negative events alike. The Life Experiences Survey described by Sarason, Johnson, and Siegel (see supplemental readings) attempts to improve change measurement by asking subjects to rate each life event on a seven-point scale, ranging from extremely negative to extremely positive impact. Students will be interested in the content of the following ten items that Sarason et al. added just for college students:

a. Beginning a new school experience at a higher academic level (college, graduate school, professional school, etc.)
b. Changing to a new school at same academic level (undergraduate, graduate, etc.)
c. Academic probation
d. Being dismissed from dormitory or other residence
e. Failing an important exam
f. Changing a major
g. Failing a course
h. Dropping a course
i. Joining a fraternity or sorority
j. Financial problems concerning school (in danger of not having sufficient money to continue)

4. Set up a demonstration of biofeedback to reduce muscle tension in the neck or to lower blood pressure. This makes an engaging introduction to the use of this technique with various psychosomatic disorders. Technical equipment and sophistication are required for this demonstration but, if available, the educational benefits are well worth the difficulties.

Supplemental Readings

See the December, 1982, issue of the *Journal of Consulting and Clinical Psychology* for a review of research and treatment studies on a wide range of physical disorders in which psychological factors have been shown to play a role in etiology or response to treatment.

Friedman, M., & Rosenman, R. H. (1974). *Type A behavior and your heart*. New York: Knopf. This is an early collection of research on the Type A type, written for a general audience. Too long to be assigned to students, selected parts may make good supplemental reading or lecture material.

Goleman, D. (1976, August). Migraine and tension headaches. *Psychology Today*, 41–42. This is a general survey of what is known about migraine and tension headaches. It shows how the problem is not in the brain but in the flow of blood. The author argues that relaxation and aspirin are still the best treatments, although biofeedback is promising.

James, S., Hartnett, S. A., & Kalsbeek, W. A. (1983). John Henryism and blood pressure differences among black men. *Journal of Behavioral Medicine, 6,* 259—268. "John Henryism" is Sherman James's term for a personality style seen in men heavily committed to hard work and a "do or die" attitude toward adversity. Named after the nineteenth-century folk hero, this style is seen in many black men known to have hypertension and to be at risk for various coronary disorders. This article reports analyses of education and John Henryism as predictors of blood pressure differences among black men studied in James's recent socio-epidemiological field study of a predominantly black town in the rural South.

Sarason, I. G., Johnson, J. H., & Siegel, J. (1978). Assessing the impact of life changes: Development of the Life Experiences Survey. *Journal of Consulting and Clinical Psychology, 46,* 932—946. This article addresses problems with Holmes and Rahe's original Social Readjustment Rating Scale and reports the development of an improved approach. This is the first of several improved scales of life change to be published in recent years. With Sarason et al.'s scale, subjects rate the extent of positive and negative impact instead of simply noting whether the event occurred. In addition, ten items applicable only to college students are added at the end. (These items are listed in the third classroom demonstration suggested for this chapter.)

Films

Patterns of pain (28 minutes, Canadian Broadcasting Corp., Filmmakers Library, 133 E. 58th St., Suite 703A, New York, NY 10022). This film presents a psychologist, a physician, and a zoologist speaking about the perception of pain in the nervous system. A number of phenomena highly relevant to health psychology are discussed and illustrated: absence of pain perception in those wounded in battle, pain control through hypnosis, and surgical techniques for implanting pain-blocking electrodes.

Stress: A disease of our time (35 minutes, Time-Life Multi-Media, 100 Eisenhower Drive, Paramus, NJ 07652). This film describes the general effects of stress on people and presents illustrative research on migraine headaches, ulcers, and asthma.

Stress (11 minutes, Contemporary Films, McGraw-Hill Book Co., 1221 Ave. of the Americas, New York, NY 10020). This is a short presentation of Selye's general adaptation syndrome. Because it is so short, it can be used in toto in class.

Examination Items

IDENTIFICATION AND SHORT-ANSWER QUESTIONS

1. What are stigmata?
2. Differentiate "psychosomatic" and "somatoform" disorders.
3. What is the diathesis-stress model?
4. What is "immunologic memory"?
5. What is "explanatory style?"
6. What is a continual emergency reaction?
7. Differentiate Type A and Type B personalities.
8. Define and give examples of "voodoo death."
9. What is the general adaptation syndrome?
10. What is Holmes and Rahe's "Social Readjustment Rating Scale"?
11. What is social support, and why is it thought to be important?

ESSAY QUESTIONS

1. What is the Type A personality, and what evidence argues for and against its contribution to coronary heart disease?
2. What evidence supports the proposition that feelings of helplessness and lack of control lead to lowered immunocompetence?

CHAPTER 11

Depression and Suicide

Overview

Because every student has at some time felt sadness, had pessimistic thoughts that were self-defeating, been apathetic, and found little enjoyment in ordinary pleasures, depression is a topic of high initial interest to everyone. Some will have had family members who were clinically depressed or been impaired themselves, and a few will have had first-hand experience with suicidal thoughts, gestures, or the bewilderment that comes from knowing someone who committed suicide. Instructors can capitalize on this high relevance to students' experiences to stimulate their curiosity and motivation to learn about various research findings and therapeutic approaches.

Depression is a particularly useful topic in an abnormal psychology course because the major theoretical paradigms have so much that is important to say about these disorders. If a student leans more toward biological, psychoanalytic or cognitive explanations of psychopathology, he or she will find supportive evidence here. More importantly, students should be pushed to examine, resolve, and integrate competing theories.

Sample Lecture Outline

The lecture outline presented below is a straightforward, information-oriented coverage of the material with optional discussion probes included at several points. Several discussion-oriented experiences to stimulate student thinking can be included in this lecture in place of whatever material instructors choose to omit. The biological and cognitive models of depression have added so much to our understanding of depression in recent years that it will be extremely difficult to cover the wealth of material in this chapter in less than two fifty-minute class meetings. The outline that follows assumes that three class meetings have been scheduled for this topic.

1. Stimulate students' curiosity about depression by showing how common it is and pointing out how much contemporary research models have added

to our knowledge in recent years. Make the incidence figures concrete by pointing out how many people in the room can be expected to have known someone with depressive symptoms or to have experienced these symptoms themselves. This is a good place to mention briefly the risk factors associated with depression, especially the greater incidence of symptoms in women, persons from different birth cohorts, and people who have suffered a loss and stress. If you wish to focus on these vulnerability concerns, have students speculate on why these patterns have occurred.

2. Describe the four types of depressive symptoms and point out how a deficit in *any* of these areas of functioning can cause problems in the others. You may also wish to get students to draw out these relationships by asking, "How do all these symptom clusters influence one another?" or "How could all come from a common source?"

3. Differentiate the two major types of depression (unipolar and bipolar) and show how these terms are an improvement over such older terms as "manic-depressive psychosis" and "involutional melancholia." Instructors who also want to mention the endogenous-exogenous distinction to juxtapose biological and learning explanations of causation should note the recent evidence limiting the usefulness of this traditional distinction.

4. Emphasize one of the most puzzling facts about depression: the regularity and self-limiting nature of the symptoms across cultures. Preview the three theoretical models of depression to be covered in the next meeting, indicating they are very important and will shed considerable light on some of the mysteries of this disorder.

Introduce the models by saying a few words about why several are needed and how they are not necessarily mutually exclusive.

5. When introducing the *biological model*, emphasize the obvious dependence of behavior and experience on biology and that we know certain parts of the brain have a powerful effect on reward and punishment. Psychology students know this intellectually, but encouraging them to appreciate the importance of the brain helps them take the biological model more seriously.

Then go into the catecholamine hypothesis. Pointing to Figure 11-3 in the text will help give everyone a quick review of the way impulses are transmitted over nerve synapses; many students will need this. As you explain the evidence supporting this hypothesis, point out that it is common in biological research in psychopathology to integrate what is learned from studies of neurotransmitters in the brains of animals with what is known about the use of psychotropic drugs in humans. Be sure to emphasize that total norepinephrine activity will be increased by a reduction in breakdown or reuptake.

Mention briefly the biological treatments and give students a chance to ask questions about them. Many will have questions about ECT, and some may use political arguments to attack its use. Some may mention the movement to limit its use by municipal ordinance in Berkeley. A good response to their understandable concerns is to ask how else they would treat a severely depressed individual who has not responded to other treatment methods and who requires tube and intravenous feeding to stay alive. Point out that although ECT is not pretty, it is often preferable in cases where a person's life is at stake.

6. Point out that the *psychoanalytic model* is most useful for accounting for why a given individual developed depression as a response to stress. If you wish, mention briefly the three parts of the psychoanalytic explanation presented in the text, but do not spend a great deal of time on them unless you wish to emphasize the psychodynamic model. If you want to stimulate discussion on this model, focus on the case presented in the text and ask, "How would you use other models to account for the woman's story?"

7. Put the *cognitive model* in perspective by pointing out how contemporary the Beck and learned helplessness formulations are. A good way to begin is to present a clinical example illustrating logical errors, arbitrary inference, overgeneralization, etc., and ask students to point out these concepts. This will produce high involvement, as well as giving students an opportunity to apply cognitive concepts. Beck's depressive triad is straightforward and needs little elaboration, but the learned helplessness paradigm —especially its relevance to clinical depression—will be more difficult for students to grasp. Spending some time on the comparison presented in Table 11-1 should help. Students will better appreciate the cognitive model if the effective therapeutic methods following from it are clear. Emphasize the provocative results of the major study of therapy for depression reported in the text.

8. Help students evaluate the three models of depression by pointing out how they focus on different symptom clusters (biological on physical symptoms, cognitive on thoughts, etc.) and emphasizing that none accounts for other symptoms well. Also mention that none of the theories can predict *which* individuals will become depressed nor account for the well-documented self-limiting nature of unipolar depression.

9. Introduce *bipolar depression* by reviewing the differences between bipolar and unipolar depression, especially differences in epidemiology and family patterns. You may then want to describe manic symptoms and ask students to describe persons they have known who show them. Their descriptions are likely to provide examples of how manic symptoms, when controlled, can lead to creativity and achievement. Point out that the effectiveness of lithium treatment and the strength of genetic patterns argue more for the biological model of this less common form of depressive symptomatology.

10. Because everyone is fascinated with self-inflicted death, you can count on students to read the suicide section closely on their own. Other than

reviewing the mythology around suicide, there is little essential content to be presented. Thus, if time becomes scarce, this topic may be touched on only briefly. If time is available, however, it is a particularly useful topic for discussion. Suicide is so interesting to students and raises so many issues for society that they will respond well to queries such as, "Do individuals have a right to take their own lives?" or "Should medical personnel help terminally ill patients who request it to end their lives?"

Demonstrations

1. Give students a concrete example of depression and ask why they believe the person felt and behaved as he or she did. This can be done by describing the case of a depressed patient in some detail, especially one you have worked with personally. Bringing in a video or audio tape of a short interview segment will help as well, even if it is role played rather than actual. Five minutes of taped material is sufficient. Be sure to allow more time for the discussion afterward than for the actual observation.

2. Instruct students during the preceding class meeting to take the selected items from the Beck Depression Inventory in Box 11-2 and bring in their scores. Tally their anonymous scores on the board and ask, "How can we account for differences among college students on a simple scale like this?" Be a devil's advocate in the resulting discussion to help them appreciate more fully the advantages and limitations of questionnaire approaches to research, as well as the three models of depression discussed in the text.

3. Write two lists of ten simple anagrams (e.g., "s-o-h-r-e") on the board and tell students they have thirty seconds to put each one in the correct order. Divide the class in half and assign them one of the lists. Make the lists identical except for the order of the anagrams. Begin with two impossible problems (e.g., "t-a-d-c-r") on one list and end with them on the other. Pretest your problems to be sure they are not too easy or difficult, i.e., the typical student should be able to solve them in thirty seconds. Keep time as the group works and instruct them to go on to the next one after each thirty seconds. Tell them not to go back to unfinished problems. After putting up the correct answers, ask students in the different groups to report how many they got correct and discuss how they felt as they worked on them. You are likely to replicate the learned helplessness phenomenon in which having the impossible problem first leads to less motivation on subsequent ones.

Supplemental Readings

Beck, A. T., & Kovacs, M. (1977, January). A new fast therapy for depression. *Psychology Today*, 94–102. This highly readable article presents Beck's cognitive view of depression and cognitive therapy. The authors discuss ways to help individuals pinpoint their unrealistic expectancies and misinterpretations of themselves and others.

Freud, S. (1917). Mourning and Melancholia. In J. Strachey (Ed. and Trans.), *The complete psychological works* (Vol. 14). New York: Norton, 1976. Freud's classic paper on depression.

Klerman, G. L. (1979, April). The age of melancholy? *Psychology Today*, 36–42. A general article supporting the proposition that depression has replaced anxiety as the major concern of contemporary society. The author hypothesizes that this may have resulted from a growing lack of connectedness with other people and institutions and feelings of powerlessness in the face of social change.

Koro, T., & Ohara, K. (1973, March). Morita therapy. *Psychology Today*, 63–68. This article describes a form of psychotherapy developed in 1920 by a Japanese therapist, Masatake Morita. It is a highly structured inpatient approach that moves through four phases, beginning with total bed rest for several days and progressing to life skill training that stresses active work and responsibility for behavior.

Lewinsohn, P. M., & Libert, J. (1972). Pleasant events, activity schedules and depression. *Journal of Abnormal Psychology, 79,* 291–295. This early behavioral study of depression found support for the association between the number of pleasant events subjects report and their mood. These data are interpreted as supporting the relationship between rate of positive reinforcement and intensity of depression.

Scarf, M. (1977, April). The more sorrowful sex. *Psychology Today*, 44–52. A thoughtful article addressing the large differences in rates of depression between men and women. Cultural expectations and differences in desires for bondedness with others are considered as contributing factors.

Seiden, R. (1966). Campus tragedy: A study of student suicide. *Journal of Abnormal and Social Psychology, 7,* 389–399. Twenty-three college students who committed suicide are compared with the general student population on age, major, and academic standing. Because it is about college students, it is useful as supplemental reading or as a source for data to be included in lecture.

Seligman, M. E. P., et al. (1979). Depressive attributional style. *Journal of Abnormal Psychology, 88,* 242–247. A good research article for students to read and critique. It presents results of a study of 145 undergraduates who rated various situations according to three attributions related to whether helplessness produces depression. Support for the three attributional dimensions was found.

Shneidman, E. S. (1970, August). The enemy. *Psychology Today*, 37–41. This renowned student of death explores the role of death in the thoughts and behavior of living men and women. He argues that coming to grips with death is a good means to attaining life.

Films

A case of suicide (30 minutes, Time-Life Films, 100 Eisenhower Drive, Paramus, NJ 07652). This film shows the story of a seventeen-year-old mother who committed suicide. Various causes of her death are considered.

Depression: A study of abnormal behavior (26 minutes, CRM Educational Films, P.O. Box 641, Del Mar, CA 92014). A particularly interesting case of agitated depression is examined from varying theoretical perspectives.

One man's madness (32 minutes, Time-Life Multi-Media, 100 Eisenhower Drive, Paramus, NJ 07652). Documentary of a writer who developed manic-depressive disorder. His progressive alienation and withdrawal are documented as his mood swings between the extremes of ecstasy and severe depression.

Suicide clinic: A cry for help (28 minutes, Audio-Visual Center, Indiana University, Bloomington, IN 47401). Demonstrates the variability of people who attempt suicide and how suicide prevention clinics try to be accessible to those in danger.

Examination Items

IDENTIFICATION AND SHORT-ANSWER QUESTIONS
1. Differentiate endogenous and exogenous depression.
2. What is the "catecholamine hypothesis?"
3. Differentiate the biological mechanisms of MAO inhibiting and tricyclic antidepressant medications.
4. How did Freud distinguish between normal mourning and depression?
5. What is the cognitive triad?
6. What is reattribution training?
7. What are the major techniques of cognitive therapy for depression?
8. What are the symptoms of mania?
9. What is "late luteal phase disphoric disorder?"
10. How is lithium used in the treatment of affective disorders?
11. Differentiate anomic, egoistic, and altruistic suicide.

ESSAY QUESTIONS

1. Discuss the four major clusters of depressive symptoms, showing how they can affect one another.

2. Discuss how unipolar and bipolar affective disorders are similar and different. What justification is there for the belief that they may come from different sources?

3. Who in our society is most vulnerable to depression?

4. Define and give examples of the five logical errors Beck believes characterize depressive thinking.

5. Describe the essential research paradigm for learned helplessness experiments with humans and animals.

6. Discuss how the internal-external, stable-unstable, and global-specific dimensions influence how an individual may respond to an uncontrollable frustration.

7. How similar is the behavior of individuals in learned helplessness experiments and those showing clinical depression?

8. Discuss the limitations of the cognitive model of depression.

9. What are some common misconceptions about suicide, and why are they believed to be incorrect?

CHAPTER 12

The Schizophrenias

Overview

Instructors can count on students to have both high initial interest in schizophrenia, as well as many inaccurate assumptions and unrealistic attitudes about it. They will all have been exposed to distortions in the popular press, on television, and in the movies about "schizos," weirdos with split personalities who are dangerous to others as well as themselves. Even when popular misconceptions have been dispatched, this high interest can be used to help students learn the wealth of clinical and research information known about this disorder. Because it offers the strongest evidence to date for the importance of genetic predispositions to adult psychopathology, even students most committed to psychodynamic or behavioral models will have to give the biomedical perspective serious attention here.

There are five basic topics that need to be covered in some detail: (1) myths and definitional criteria, (2) types and dimensions, (3) symptoms, (4) causes, and (5) treatments of schizophrenia. Because of the quantity of important material to be covered, at least two classes will be needed for this chapter. The sample outline assumes that two classes will be used and devotes special attention to the various symptoms and etiological models. The supplementary readings, films, and demonstrations are designed to maintain interest and flesh out student understanding by giving them specific examples to consider.

A major objective for this chapter should be to remove some of the mystification surrounding schizophrenia. Even though fascinated by the bizarreness and extreme symptoms of this disorder, most students will think of schizophrenics as somehow different, as sharing few characteristics with themselves. As much as you can, help students to empathize with schizophrenics, to imagine what it's like to be unable to control one's thoughts and emotions and to be almost as perplexed by one's internal experiences as by the world outside. If students are able to see much schizophrenic language and motor behavior as highly disguised attempts to communicate, they are more likely to see schizophrenics as persons.

Sample Lecture Outline

1. Begin by asking, "How many of you have ever seen a schizophrenic?" Get students to describe those they have seen before and ask: "What makes you think they fit this classification?" An opening discussion such as this provides a good introduction to the first points to be made about the history and mythology surrounding schizophrenia. Acknowledge that students— especially those who have not had sufficient first-hand contact with schizophrenics—are likely to have unrealistic expectancies about schizophrenics, implicit beliefs that can be questioned as this topic is considered.

2. The DSM-III-R definitional criteria need to be stressed, especially the distinction between *temporal* and *substantive* criteria. Tell students that this distinction is a change from the definition in DSM-II, which allowed a short-term, acute episode to be classified as schizophrenia. Stress that a disturbance in *thoughts* most characterizes persons showing the disorder, although perceptions, emotions, and behaviors are also commonly affected as well.

3. Focus next on the important dimensions along which schizophrenics vary, especially the newer distinction between Type I and Type II schizophrenia around which many of the research findings reported in the text are organized. Emphasize that this dimension may point the way to a major etiological difference in the kind of biological predispositions among the various individuals.

4. In dealing with the symptoms of schizophrenia, emphasize the research findings about perceptual, thought, and affective symptoms of schizophrenia, as well as how they show themselves clinically. The laboratory research presented in the text on hallucinations, attention, and overinclusive or distracted thinking provides excellent illustrations of how psychological methods can be usefully applied to this major form of psychopathology.

5. A good way to bring the first class to a close is to ask students to imagine how they might react were they to find their perceptions or thinking process changing with no plausible explanation. Encourage them to view some schizophrenic symptoms—especially the accessory symptoms of suspiciousness, grandiosity, hostility-belligerence, and resistiveness-uncooperativeness —as not unreasonable reactions to the experience of finding thoughts and perceptions to be disordered.

6. Of the four main etiological theories to be considered (genetic, neurotransmitter, family communication, and social), research supporting the genetic and neurotransmitter hypotheses is most important. Begin with the genetic approach, making certain that students appreciate the implication of the consistent differences found in concordance rates between MZ and DZ twins, especially Gottesman and Shields's study showing the difference

to be even greater for chronics, and in incidence between parents and siblings. Help students fully understand the logic of the experiments by asking, "Even though these twin and family incidence studies have amazingly consistent results, can we conclude that schizophrenia is genetic in origin?" The ensuing discussion will help lay a foundation for the adoption studies.

7. By this point, students should be well prepared to appreciate the significance of the adoption and at-risk children studies, and that a genetic predisposition is necessary but not sufficient for most cases of schizophrenia to develop. Stress that the predisposition is probably not a simple qualitative propensity but rather dimensions associated with emotional sensitivity and looseness of thinking. These dimensions may be essential for creativity and high achievement for many, although associated with dysfunction for others. Paul Meehl's classic article on genetic predisposition (see supplemental readings) can be summarized here with good effect.

8. The dopamine hypothesis is still one of the strongest explanations in abnormal psychology, and it is important that students understand it well and appreciate its potential importance for future understanding of brain processes as well as Type I schizophrenia. Although the specific facts are presented clearly in the text, spend some time going over the basics (clinical effects and side effects of phenothiazine treatment, amphetamine abuse, Parkinson's disease, and studies of biochemical action in animals) to be sure students understand these various types of supporting evidence. This hypothesis illustrates scientific process in psychopathology well and lays the foundation for one of the most important points in this chapter: Many of the symptoms shown by schizophrenics could result from a common attentional deficit that is biological and likely genetic in origin.

9. If sufficient time remains, spend a minute or so on a robust finding concerning the epidemiology of schizophrenia: It is strongly inversely related to social class. Mention the social selection and social stress explanations of this pattern. The results of the Dohrenwend and Dohrenwend study cited in the supplemental readings offer an excellent way to illustrate these two opposing hypotheses.

10. Conclude the topic of schizophrenia by briefly addressing treatment. Drugs are the major topic here and although they need not be gone into in detail, students should appreciate their power to control the fundamental symptoms of schizophrenia. Mention their drawbacks, to be sure, but do not downplay the fact that they are a major advance in the treatment of schizophrenia and of far greater effectiveness than any form of psychotherapy yet developed. Emphasize that treatment is even better when drugs are combined with other psychogenic treatments to offset the secondary effects of this major form of psychopathology.

Demonstrations

1. Demonstrate the importance of knowing the history of a schizophrenic's life and the context of his or her symptoms when making a diagnosis and estimate of prognosis by giving students written case studies of an individual showing an acute episode much like the case of Carl presented in the text. Give half the class a version that mentions the precipitating stresses in the person's life and omit this information from the description given the others. Ask everyone to rate the patient on the degree to which his or her symptoms indicate the presence of schizophrenia and the probability that he or she will regain full functioning after treatment. Have students in the two groups hand in their ratings (or report them verbally if you take time to tally them in class) before revealing the different information. What the resulting data are almost certain to reveal is the moderating effect on diagnosis and prognosis of background information on precipitating stress.

2. Demonstrate the tendency of schizophrenics to be overinclusive in their associations by reading students the following items from a test used to measure this phenomena (see the Rattan and Chapman citation under the supplemental readings) and asking them to write down the correct answer:

1. "Pool" means the same as
    a. puddle
    b. notebook
    c. swim
    d. none of the above
2. "Shoot" means the same as
    a. rifle
    b. rug
    c. sprout
    d. none of the above
3. "Scale" means the same as
    a. pin
    b. fish
    c. climb
    d. none of the above
4. "Police" means the same as
    a. arrest
    b. drop
    c. keep in order
    d. none of the above
5. "Ape" means the same as
    a. hairy
    b. ball
    c. imitate or copy
    d. none of the above

6. "Duck" means the same as
   a. swim
   b. quack
   c. lower head suddenly
   d. none of the above

3. Read a few passages relating conversations between schizophrenics and ask students to interpret the meaning in the conversations. Ask, "What might these persons be saying to each other?" Pages 93—97 of Haley's *Strategies of Psychotherapy* (see supplemental readings) and numerous sections in Rokeach's *Three Christs of Ypsilanti* provide examples from which to choose.

4. Make a videotape showing a family interacting around a dining room table at mealtime or in a group interview in a clinician's office. Have the family members illustrate the types of communication distortion discussed in the text: injection of meaning, concealing clear meaning, and denial of meaning. Student volunteers can be recruited to role play a family in class or before video cameras for later use. After the demonstration, ask students to react to what they saw in the communication of this "schizophrenogenic family" before showing how the simulated interaction illustrated common communication problems found in families with a schizophrenic member. If this demonstration is used, mention the results of the Liem study cited in the following section which show that schizophrenics tend to bring out distorted communications from others, even parents of non-schizophrenic children.

Supplemental Readings

Dohrenwend, B. P., & Dohrenwend, B. S. (1972). Psychiatric epidemiology: An analysis of "true prevalence" studies. In S. Golann & C. Eisdorfer (Eds.), *Handbook of community mental health*. New York: Appleton-Century-Crofts. Studies of psychiatric epidemiology are surveyed as a lengthy introduction to a critical comparison of the social stress and social selection hypotheses into the robust inverse association between schizophrenia and SES. The psychiatric incidence of our groups of lower SES subjects were compared: Blacks, Puerto Ricans, Jews, and Irish. The Dorhenwends argue that the incidence figures should be *lower* for the two groups of racial minorities if the social selection hypothesis is correct (because discrimination would keep the genetic talent in these two groups from rising to its appropriate level) and *higher* if the social stress position is correct. Mixed support for the social stress position was found.

Haley, J. (1963). *Strategies of psychotherapy*. New York: Grune & Stratton. The author argues that relationship communication complexities have a powerful effect on psychotherapy. Pages 93–97 present an analysis of a conversation between two schizophrenics showing the meaningfulness of their seemingly "crazy" language.

Liem, J. (1974). Effects of verbal communications of parents and children: A comparison of normal and schizophrenic families. *Journal of Consulting and Clinical Psychology, 42,* 438–450. This study compared communication clarity in mother-father-child triads. The clever design first examined communication clarity in a group of triads in which the child was schizophrenic, comparing them to the interactions of a group of parents interacting with their normal child. Then the children switched parents and communication was again studied, except the parents of a schizophrenic talked with a non-schizophrenic child and the parents of normal children talked with a schizophrenic. The results showed that the parents of normal children tended to show the same kinds of unclear communications when talking with a schizophrenic as did the parents of a schizophrenic.

Maher, B. A. (1968, November). The shattered language of schizophrenia. *Psychology Today,* 30–33. Discusses the "cipher" and "avoidance" hypotheses about the functions of disjointed schizophrenic language and attempts to identify the psycholinguistic "rules" of schizophrenic speech by constructing examples of schizophrenic and non-schizophrenic language and subjecting them to linguistic analysis.

Meehl, P. (1962). Schizotaxia, schizotypy, and schizophrenia. *American Psychologist, 17,* 827–838. This is a classic article on the genetic predisposition to schizophrenia. It is still one of the most persuasive theoretical presentations of the position that a genetically acquired underlying personality pattern, under stress, can lead to schizophrenia.

Rabkin, J. G. (1979). Criminal behavior and discharged mental patients. *Psychological Bulletin, 86,* 1–27. The author reviews a great deal of research and concludes that discharged mental patients have higher arrest records than non-patients *only* if the patients had previous arrest records. In the studies surveyed, patients without previous arrests never had higher and sometimes had lower arrest records than non-patients.

Rattan, R., & Chapman, J. P. (1973). Associative intrusions in schizophrenic verbal behavior. *Journal of Abnormal Psychology, 82,* 169–173. Two multiple-choice vocabulary tests were developed, one form containing words with strong associations as incorrect alternatives. After pretesting to be sure the forms were of comparable intellectual difficulty, the performance of chronic schizophrenics on the two tests was compared to that of normals. The schizophrenics showed significantly poorer performance on the items containing incorrect associations. (See classroom demonstration 2 for an illustration of the items with distracting associations.)

Films

Breakdown (40 minutes, McGraw-Hill Textfilms, 110 15th St., Del Mar, CA 92014). This depicts an actual case of a schizophrenic woman, showing her outpatient and inpatient treatment and follow-up. This is a good portrayal of the typical course of the disorder, including a positive return to family living.

The McGraw-Hill (110 156th St., Del Mar, CA 92014) "Mental Symptoms" series is excellent. *Schizophrenia—Catatonic type* (12 minutes), *Schizophrenia—Hebephrenic type* (13 minutes), and *Schizophrenia—Simple type* (11 minutes) are all useful clinical portrayals.

Schizophrenia: The shattered mirror (60 minutes, Audio-Visual Center, Division of University Extension, Indiana University, Bloomington, IN 47401). This film shows the institutional care and case history of a schizophrenic young man. Current research is nicely integrated with this engaging portrait.

A true madness (35 minutes, Time-Life Films, Inc., 43 W. 16th St., New York, NY 10011). This film uses conversations between schizophrenics and their physicians to illustrate the variability and common features of this disorder.

Examination Items

IDENTIFICATION AND SHORT-ANSWER QUESTIONS
1. Define "dementia praecox."
2. What was Adolph Meyer's view of schizophrenia?
3. Differentiate the temporal and substantive criteria for diagnosing schizophrenia.
4. What are delusions?
5. What are hallucinations?
6. What are the symptoms of the paranoid schizophrenic?
7. What are the symptoms of the disorganized schizophrenic?
8. What are the symptoms of the catatonic schizophrenic?
9. Differentiate Type I and Type II schizophrenia.
10. What are clang associations?
11. What are neologisms?
12. What is overinclusiveness?
13. Differentiate delusions of grandeur, control, persecution, and reference.
14. What is a proband?
15. Define "concordant."
16. What are schizophrenogenic families?

17. Differentiate expressed emotion and communication deviance in communications of families with schizophrenic members.
18. What should be included in a program of milieu therapy for schizophrenics?

ESSAY QUESTIONS

1. What are some common myths about schizophrenics and why are they false?
2. Describe the Type I–Type II dimension of schizophrenia and what it is thought to represent.

(Note: Students may be asked to answer all three or only some of the next three questions.)

3. Discuss the following category of schizophrenic symptoms: perceptual difficulties.
4. Discuss the following category of schizophrenic symptoms: thought disorders.
5. Discuss the following category of schizophrenic symptoms: affective disturbances.
6. Discuss the evidence that there is a genetic predisposition for schizophrenia.
7. State the dopamine hypothesis and discuss the evidence supporting it.

Sexual Behavior, Dysfunction, and Disorder

Overview

Students will be quite interested in the next two chapters, especially Chapter 13 on sex. Instructors can be sure this chapter will be read carefully and when assigned (if not earlier!). High involvement also means overinvolvement for some students. Some students will have troubling personal questions about their sexual functioning or identity and may have elected to take this course primarily to have them answered. Therefore, in addition to mastering content, appropriate objectives are to give students an opportunity to ask personal questions, reassure them their sexual fantasies or acts are not unusual or "bad," and, if appropriate, direct them to professional counselors. Instructors need do little to stimulate student involvement and motivation to learn the factual details. Clarifying text content, answering questions, and leading discussion on attitudes will usually suffice to produce solid achievement and memorable class sessions.

Because students will learn much of the content on their own, the topics in this chapter *can* be covered briefly in a single class meeting. Students will be disappointed that more time was not spent on one of their favorite topics, however, and allocating two classes, one for sexual function and dysfunction and one for sexual disorders, is a better approach.

Sample Lecture Outline

1. Begin by noting the shift from disorders with a strong individual focus to an interpersonal group in which other persons are more involved. Point out that people frequently have strong emotional or judgmental beliefs about these disorders, that the influence of personal values and attitudes is stronger here than for any disorders studied in the course. Encourage students to examine their own attitudes in light of what they will be learning.

2. Introduce our current knowledge of sexual physiology by crediting the pioneering research of Kinsey and Masters and Johnson. Outline the various changes occurring in the erotic arousal and desire, physical excitement, and orgasm phases of the human sexual response and ask if students have questions before moving on. Do not be surprised if students are slower to respond to requests for questions or discussion than usual. Stress the amazing similarity of sexual response across individuals and between men and women and point out that the overwhelming proportion of sexual dysfunctions results from learned anxiety which interferes with the body's functioning.

3. Briefly list the dysfunctions covered in the text (arousal, erectile, and orgasmic dysfunctions and premature ejaculation) and allow students to ask for clarification. The direct sexual treatment commonly used for each of these disorders can be mentioned briefly, as they are described as an additional stimulus for student questions. Avoid spending a great deal of class time describing these dysfunctions.

4. Theories about the causes of sexual dysfunctions need more coverage. Point out that the psychodynamic and behavioral theories share an assumption that learned anxiety interferes with the body's ability to function sexually. They differ in how they formulate the source of that anxiety: psychoanalysts assume unconscious conflicts are at work and behaviorists assume learned associations are the cause. Stress that Masters and Johnson's basic research and direct treatment methods have done more to offer hope for sexually dysfunctional individuals than either theory.

5. Bring the discussion of direct sexual therapy to a close by evaluating it. Ask, "Even though Masters and Johnson's work is clearly a major breakthrough, what is wrong with it? What are problems with this approach?" Students will cite the limitations mentioned in the book about how outcome data are reported, but they may also offer other limitations. If they do not raise them, however, emphasize that these approaches work best within the context of stable relationships in which partners are committed to improving and can communicate minimally with each other. Also point out that some authorities object to the use of active behavioral treatments on moral grounds (see Bailey's, Wagner's, and Wilson's responses to Zeiss's article as referenced under the supplemental readings).

6. Address the issue of social values and sexuality. A primary topic to be focused on is homosexuality and the fact that only the ego-dystonic type is still considered a legitimate topic for a course in abnormal psychology. Some instructors may choose to deal with homosexuality more generally out of a commitment to undo the mental health profession's past transgressions toward homosexuals, to help students recognize gay persons as just like themselves save one small distinction, and to encourage students to be less fearful of their homophobia. If homosexuality is dealt with in detail, remember (and remind the class) that some people in the class are attracted to

members of the same sex and avoid trying to convince the class that they should adopt the instructor's personal values. Do not be surprised if students find it very hard to talk about this topic in the usual discussion format. The suggested readings, demonstrations, and exercises can be used to help sensitize students to their own values here.

7. Students will be much more open about their interest in the paraphilias than about homosexuality. Present a case study—someone you have seen professionally, if possible—to illustrate and contrast the psychodynamic and behavioral views of cause and treatment. This will open up the class to discussion after the inhibiting effect of dealing with homosexuality. Instructors might ask, "Now that the mental health professions have said there is nothing necessarily abnormal about sexual behavior between members of the same sex, why should they still say it is not normal to receive sexual pleasure from pornography, fetishes, transvestism, or sadomasochism among consenting adults?" This discussion can highlight political and value differences in the class and clarify the criteria practicing clinicians actually use. Davidson's 1978 article (see the supplemental readings) on the ethical responsibilities of clinicians *not* to treat homosexuals for their sexual preference can also be used here to stimulate student discussion and examination of their attitudes. Note that the case presented in the *SuperShrink* computer interview simulation involves exhibitionism. If the *SuperShrink* laboratory is assigned, the case portrayed there provides an excellent vehicle with which to contrast psychodynamic and cognitive-behavioral perspectives of the paraphilias.

8. If there is time, focus on transsexuality. This topic can be approached from an ethical perspective ("Should society allow transsexuals to have access to surgery and hormone treatment to change their sexual anatomy?") or from a developmental/physiological perspective, using the research cited in the text on drug-produced cases of hermaphroditism.

Demonstrations

1. Invite an openly homosexual person (a male and a female if available) to speak to your class and answer questions. Many campuses have gay students organizations that offer speakers. This is a good way to help students question their assumptions, although it will take more class time than instructors may want to devote to homosexuality.

2. An alternative method of accomplishing many of the same goals is to ask for student volunteers to interview some gay persons (persons they know or the instructor finds for them) and share their experiences with the class. Encourage them to ask how being gay is different and not different from being "straight," when the persons first became aware of their preference,

and how others react when they find out about it. Instructors may also ask local gay students about organizing a visit to a gay bar and then accompany any of the class who wish to go. Each of these options requires discussion afterward for maximum learning and attitude change.

3. Construct a survey of student sexual attitudes. Have the class take it and distribute it to other students to complete and return anonymously to the instructor. Compare these local responses to the published data. The survey reported by Bauman and Wilson (see the supplemental readings) lists normative data for college student samples in 1968 and 1972. It can easily be replicated within your class.

Supplemental Readings

Bauman, K. E., & Wilson, R. R. (1976). Premarital attitudes of unmarried university students: 1968 vs. 1972. *Archives of Sexual Behavior, 5,* 327–333. The authors present comparative data on college students' attitudes toward petting and sexual intercourse in relationships of varying intensity and commitment. Useful for comparison to data collected by your students.

Boswell, J. (1980). *Christianity, social tolerance, and homosexuality: Gay people in Western Europe from the beginning of the Christian Era to the Fourteenth Century.* Chicago: University of Chicago Press. Boswell traces the course of contemporary prejudice and persecution of gay people. He convincingly makes the case that social intolerance predated the emphasis in Christian dogma on the special sin of homosexuality. This is a magnificent scholarly essay by a medieval historian, but one that is more useful for background information than for reading by students.

Davidson, G. C. (1978). Not can but ought: The treatment of homosexuality. *Journal of Consulting and Clinical Psychology, 46,* 165–169. This article is based on Davidson's controversial speech to the Association for the Advancement of Behavior Therapy in which he advocated a discontinuation of behavior therapy for homosexuals wishing to change their sexual orientation, even when they seek it. His thesis is that therapists are supporting repressive social attitudes by treating the victims of those prejudices.

Montagu, A. (1978, August). A "Kinsey Report" on homosexualities. *Psychology Today, 91,* 62–66. This article surveys the wide variation in homosexual practice and preference. The data presented make the point that there is as much variability in the sexual behavior of homosexuals as in that of heterosexuals.

Zeiss, A. M., Rosen, G. M., & Zeiss, R. A. (1977). Orgasm during intercourse: A treatment strategy for women. *Journal of Consulting and Clinical Psychology, 45,* 891–895. The authors report a technique for women unable to have orgasms during intercourse. In the early stages, it teaches women to have fantasies of intercourse while masturbating. A male partner and a dildo are brought into the masturbation sessions later. Then as the women gradually approach having an orgasm, an erect penis is inserted. The graphic treatment regimen reported in this article stimulated considerable debate in a later issue of this journal (1978, *46*, 1502–1514). Kent Baily responded by raising strong objections to Zeiss et al.'s practice of teaching women to masturbate and to use dildos. He argued that such therapists were trying to change traditional values and might create later problems in women put under pressure to achieve orgasm. Nathaniel Wagner responded by arguing that Baily's objections were thinly veiled attempts to rationalize an anti-quated prejudice against masturbation. Not to let the debate rest, G. Terence Wilson responded by supporting the value of programs like that reported by Zeiss et al. if conducted with sensitivity and respect for clients' values. The Baily, Wagner, and Wilson commentaries offer a vivid example of how the personal values of psychologists affect how therapies are judged.

Films

Select films about sex and sex therapy with caution. Some good films from a few years ago—*Some of your best friends*, University of Southern California, a film from the 1960s about homosexuality—are now dated. Others may be so graphic and unnecessarily provocative as to be offensive. Some students and instructors may like a given film and others may react strongly against it. Nonetheless, here are three suggestions.

I am not this body (28 minutes, Erickson Educational Foundation, P.O. Box 185, Kendall Post Office, Miami, FL 33156). This film presents inter-views with two transsexuals: a woman who has just had sex-change surgery and a man about to undergo it. Each discusses their reasons for choosing this drastic step and illustrates the long-standing nature of transsexuals' sexual identities.

Lavander (16 minutes, Perennial Education, Inc., 477 Roger Williams Ave., P.O. Box 855 Ravinia, Highland Park, IL 60035). This film presents a warm interview between a lesbian couple. As the women describe their life together, it is apparent that theirs is an enjoyable and satisfying emotional relationship, not a popular stereotype.

Word is out (45 minutes, Mariposa Film Group, New Yorker Films, 16 W. 61st St., New York, NY 10023). This is a film portrayal of oral history inter-views with approximately 200 gay men and women from all over the country. This 45-minute version of the longer 130-minute film of the same name is a very honest, warm, and well-balanced film, probably the best film to date on homosexuals. The variety and essential humanness of the persons por-trayed rings loud and true.

Examination Items

IDENTIFICATION AND SHORT-ANSWER QUESTIONS

1. Differentiate sexual dysfunctions and disorders.
2. Differentiate erotic arousal, physical excitement, and orgasm.
3. Define "sexual unresponsiveness."
4. Differentiate primary, secondary, situation specific, and global erectile dysfunction.
5. What is "bypassing?"
6. What is premature ejaculation?
7. What is the psychodynamic explanation of a man's inability to attain an erection?
8. What factors influence the frequency of premarital intercourse in a culture?
9. Differentiate exclusive homosexuality and bisexuality.
10. Differentiate gender role and gender identity.
11. Define "paraphilia."
12. Define "fetish."
13. Differentiate transsexualism and transvestism.
14. Differentiate sadism and masochism.
15. What are the behavior and personality characteristics of exhibitionists?
16. Define "voyeurism."
17. Define "pedophile."
18. Differentiate ego-syntonic and ego-dystonic homosexuality.

ESSAY QUESTIONS

1. What are problems with survey studies of sexual behavior?
2. How are the sexual responses of men and women similar?
3. How are the types of sexual dysfunctions of men and women similar?
4. What is the behavioral explanation of sexual dysfunction in men and women?
5. How does direct sexual therapy differ from previous methods? What are its known limitations?
6. Compare and contrast the psychodynamic and behavioral views of the paraphilias.
7. How does the behavioral view explain the persistence of paraphilias?
8. What have the studies of sexual hormones and hermaphrodites given to our understanding of gender identity?

CHAPTER 14

Psychoactive Substance Use Disorders

Overview

Many students are likely to be ambivalent about the content of this chapter, especially given the conflict between the social pressures to experiment with and use psychoactive drugs and this chapter's clear presentation of the growing evidence that any drug use—from tobacco to alcohol to marijuana to stimulants to opiates—is bad for individuals and societies. For the large number of students in every class who know a close relative or friend who has a serious drug problem or who worry about their own ability to control drug use, this chapter will stimulate considerable interest and anxiety; perhaps for some, a reliving of painful childhood memories.

The chapter presents a number of recent findings about the neurophysiology of drug abuse and integrates many of them around a common conceptual formulation: the opponent-process model of addiction. General questions of why people use and become dependent on psychoactive drugs are addressed, in addition to discussing the specific characteristics of various commonly abused drugs. Underlying the complex information presented in this chapter are a number of attitudinal issues that speak directly to students' personal concerns about drug use and its associated problems. The sample lecture outline and suggested demonstrations address these attitudinal issues as well as clarifying the major points included in the text.

Sample Lecture Outline

1. Indicate that drug use and abuse is a personal question for everyone. Talk about the fact that many students have an alcoholic parent or know persons whose use of other drugs is uncontrolled and creates difficulties in their lives. Ask students to consider the paradox of drug use: For probably as long as humankind has existed, people have repeatedly put chemicals in

their bodies just to make themselves feel differently, even though they frequently feel bad later or endanger their health. Are the psychological laws governing this behavior the same as or different from other behaviors? Whether this question is asked rhetorically or students are asked to respond, indicate that today's topic will look at the general psychology of drug use as well as the forms of abnormal thoughts and behaviors resulting from various forms of drug abuse.

2. Differentiate drug *use* and *abuse*. Emphasize that abusers must show a pattern of pathological use for at least one month in which their social or occupational functioning has been impaired. Ask students to write down how many beers (or "joints") per week is likely to create a pattern of abuse. Tally their responses on the board to indicate the variability.

3. Spend enough time on the opponent-process model of addiction to be certain students understand it well and are able to apply it to common drug phenomena. The graphs included in the text will clarify their understanding and may be worth focusing on in class. However you clarify this complex model, conclude your coverage by describing various effects of specific drugs and having the class respond in Greek Chorus fashion with whether Process A or Process B is involved. Continue with this group recitation until their speed of response and accuracy are high.

4. Spend the rest of your class session(s) on the specific drugs covered, depending on your own and students' interests. Alcohol is, of course, the major drug discussed and the one most likely to be both attractive and troublesome to your students. Stress the commonalities in how empirical research—much of it biochemical and neurological—has expanded our understanding of how many commonly used drugs affect us and lead to substance abuse disorders in many individuals.

Demonstrations

1. Encourage students to organize into small teams of three or four to make some field observations of drug and alcohol use near their campus, especially where teenagers hang out. Tell them to spend a few hours there some Saturday night and pretend they are from another planet and know nothing about substance use here on Earth. Dropping in on a few bars and watching patrons leave near closing time will tell them a great deal about the role alcohol plays in many people's lives. Have teams report back to the class about what they learned.

2. Encourage students to organize into small teams of three or four to interview local police, fire, emergency transportation, and hospital emergency room personnel about how much of the human tragedy and problems they encounter in their jobs is caused by alcohol. Have these students also share what they learn with the whole class.

Supplemental Readings

Abel, E. L. (1977). The relationship between cannabis and violence: A review. *Psychological Bulletin, 84,* 193–211. The author concludes from his review that there is little unequivocal evidence relating to this issue. In general, it does *not* appear that marijuana is a cause of aggression. This conclusion is based on samples of typical users and underrepresents at-risk individuals who might react violently when under the influence of this drug, especially those with histories of violent behavior at other times.

Marlatt, G. A., Demming, B., & Reid, J. B. (1973). Loss of control drinking in alcoholics: An experimental analogue. *Journal of Abnormal Psychology, 81,* 233–241. This classic study demonstrated that the "one drink mythology" is largely an expectancy effect. Alcoholics unknowingly given alcohol primers were no more likely to drink subsequently than those not given alcohol. Also, alcoholics who believed they were given alcohol instead of the actual nonalcoholic beverage drank more than controls.

Wilson, G. T., & Lawson, D. M. (1976). Expectancies, alcohol, and sexual arousal in male social drinkers. *Journal of Abnormal Psychology, 85,* 587–594. The research reported here documents the strong effect of expectancy. Subjects believing they were drinking alcohol believed themselves to be more intoxicated than those not so persuaded.

Zinberg, N. E. (1976, December). The war over marijuana. *Psychology Today,* 44–52. The author reviews the large body of findings—marijuana is our most widely researched drug, he states—and summarizes what we do and do not know about it. Students will find the wide range of studies and variables discussed here of high interest.

Films

The perfect drug film (31 minutes, Audio-Visual Center, Indiana University, Bloomington, IN 47401). This film uses a mythical perfect drug and shows the potential effects it would have when introduced to society. It illustrates how humans have long sought a better and safer "perfect drug."

Skeszg (73 minutes, Tricontinenta Film Center, 333 6th Ave., New York, NY 10014). This film addresses the psychological and social causes of drug abuse in a hard-hitting manner. This is a long film, but it will have a strong impact on students.

Examination Items

IDENTIFICATION AND SHORT-ANSWER QUESTIONS

1. Differentiate affective pleasure, tolerance, and withdrawal.
2. What are some problems with the tension-reduction hypothesis when applied to drug abuse?
3. What is the endorphin compensation hypothesis?
4. Differentiate the pharmacological effects of alcohol and the opiates.
5. Differentiate substitution and abstinence-oriented therapy for narcotic dependence.
6. Differentiate THC and PCP and their psychological effects.

ESSAY QUESTIONS

1. What evidence supports the statement: "Alcohol is this country's number one drug problem"?
2. Discuss the opponent-process model of addiction, illustrating your points with examples from at least two of the following drugs: opiates, alcohol, stimulants, nicotine.

CHAPTER 15

Personality Disorders

Overview

Following the discussions of sexual and substance disorders, the personality disorders may seem tame to students. One way to offset this is to follow the chapter's organization and focus on the antisocial personality disorder. Psychopaths are fascinating to most people—who has not had the fantasy of being able to act impulsively with no guilt or remorse—and an in-depth discussion here lays a good foundation for Chapter 18 on legal issues. This is also a good disorder to focus on because experimental psychological research has suggested a particularly compelling and well-supported model for the biological deficit at the root of this disorder.

Although most of the class time will probably be spent on the antisocial personality disorder, do mention the other personality disorders at the beginning or the end of the class, stressing that these disorders are closest to us "normals," that they represent exaggerations of many typical personality dimensions and strategies in living. The end of Chapter 15 covers briefly eight or so of these types, and the presentation of them is clear and straightforward. Do not feel compelled to go into each of these in detail.

An overall objective for this chapter is for students to appreciate that some styles of personality functioning, taken to the extreme, can cause difficulties in living for others, even though they rarely create direct discomfort for the individual showing them. Psychopaths show the most extreme forms of such ego-syntonic disorders, but because the other categories are more likely to be closer to students' personal experience, you might use these categories to point out this essential difference between neurotic and characterological disorders.

Sample Lecture Outline

1. Begin with a case example of an antisocial, paranoid, dependent, or compulsive personality disorder. The text gives one for each type but pick another, longer case example from your own experience, from the case

books cited in the introduction to this manual, or from current news stories. After presenting the essential details, ask, "Is this individual abnormal? Why or why not?" Use the ensuing discussion to stress that the personality disorders are long-standing ego-syntonic disorders that are more troublesome to others than to the individual. Before going into the antisocial personality disorder, differentiate the personality disorders from the anxiety disorders and psychoses.

2. Put the antisocial personality disorder into perspective by touching on the historical interest in those who commit criminal acts who seem to lack the *capacity* for obeying rules and laws. Be sure students appreciate that the terms antisocial personality, psychopath, and sociopath are still used interchangeably by many professionals and researchers. In surveying this history, stimulate students' curiosity about why some individuals do not seem to become acculturated to behave like the rest of us, especially why they do not seem to develop the internal controls that make orderly civilization possible.

3. Help students learn the essential defining characteristics by comparing the system used in DSM-III-R and the more inferential criteria advocated by Cleckley. Give a few short case examples to illustrate how each system can be used and to emphasize the differences between them. Be sure to include several examples who do not fit into either system. Students should be confident in how to differentiate antisocial personalities from those persons committing impulsive or illegal acts who do not fit the criteria sufficiently to be diagnosed as sociopaths. Emphasize that only 20 to 40 percent of prison inmates, however, are likely to be classified as showing this personality style and that many psychopaths succeed in various walks of life and avoid criminal charges altogether. Cleckley's *Mask of Sanity* (see the supplemental readings) provides examples of more successful psychopaths.

4. Next go into the various types of research about the causes of this particular disorder. Of the family studies, stress Robins's (1966) important work on longitudinal predictors, indicating that this is one of the best such studies in existence. Spend most of the time on the psychological research on psychopaths' deficiencies in avoidance learning and on the other research supporting the view that they are physiologically under-aroused. Tracing the progression in evidence from Lykken's, Schachter and Latane's, and Schmauk's studies illustrates how experimental research can build on previous findings, as well as ensures that students will learn this valuable research supporting the biological deficit view. Depending on how much time remains, you may want to touch briefly on the limited research supporting a genetic basis, especially the Hutchings and Mednick adoption study described in the text.

5. This outline has covered mainly the fundamental information about the personality disorders, which can be squeezed into one seventy-five minute

class period and treated comfortably in two fifty-minute periods. If more time can be spent on the personality disorders, ask students to think about them from a *political* or *social power* perspective. Return to some of the case studies you have presented and ask, "How would a radical feminist or a Marxist view this same individual and his or her problems with others?" Because the personality disorders by definition represent difficulties with other persons, issues of power and maintenance of the social and economic status quo become highly relevant. Before devoting an entire class to this discussion, consider how you plan to treat Chapter 18 on legal issues. The discussion of personality disorders within a social context might be coordinated with how the legal issues are presented.

Demonstrations

There are several ways to give students first-hand contact with antisocial personalities and those who work with them regularly. A visit to a local prison, including group interviews with a few of the more "charming" inmates is ideal, although difficult to arrange for many. If a prison unit is nearby, inquire about this possibility. The prison may also have a community relations program that can send inmates to speak to your class. An alternative is to bring an adult or juvenile probation officer or a prison psychologist to speak to the class about examples of antisocial personalities they have seen. Any of these options will emphasize that most antisocial personalities are not as extreme in their unsympathetic behavior as the "Gary Gilmores" publicized in movies and the popular press. As with all demonstrations or visits of this type, be sure to provide time for students to process their reactions with you and each other.

Supplemental Readings

Cleckley, H. M. (1976). *The mask of sanity* (5th ed.). St. Louis: Mosby. This is the latest edition of a classic book that attempts to understand the antisocial personality by examining numerous case examples of physicians, businessmen, lawyers, scientists, psychiatrists, etc. This book provides an excellent choice of rich case examples.

Hanley, B., & Gold, M. (1973, September). The juvenile delinquent nobody knows. *Psychology Today*, 48–55. This is an engaging article on the wide range of delinquent behaviors shown by young people from all social strata and groups. Those showing these behaviors are contrasted with the small minority who actually get caught and receive what is often counterproductive treatment by the juvenile correction system.

Heilbrun, A. B. (1979). Psychopathy and violent crime. *Journal of Consulting and Clinical Psychology, 47,* 509–516. Heilbrun reports a study in which he used intelligence as a moderator of the relationship between degree of psychopathy and violent crime among a prison population. His findings suggest that the crimes of brighter psychopaths tend to be premeditated. In contrast, psychopaths of limited intelligence were more likely to commit more violent crimes.

Films

One flew over the cuckoo's nest (United Artists Entertainment, 729 7th Ave., New York, NY 10019). This is an excellent feature length film of a few years back that provides a portrait of Ken Kesey's character "McMurphy," a psychopathic individual who feigns mental illness to take a vacation from prison at a psychiatric hospital. This film is now old enough that many students may not have seen it in theaters or on television. It will provide an excellent stimulus for discussion of treatment issues, as well as presenting a reasonably accurate and highly engaging portrait of a psychopathic personality.

A psychopath (30 minutes, McGraw-Hill Films, 110 15th St., Del Mar, CA 92014). This film presents interviews with a psychiatrist, a detective, a director of rehabilitation, a prison warden, and the patient himself to reconstruct the history of a psychopathic personality. Although this film is over twenty years old, it is still useful and no comparable newer film is available.

Shotgun Joe (25 minutes, Jason Films, 2621 Palisade Ave., Riverdale, NY 10463). This is an engaging portrait of an incarcerated teenager. Various friends and acquaintances describe his good humor and leadership qualities, making a sharp contrast between Joe's own matter-of-fact description of how he got his nickname: He had a habit of clubbing victims with a sawed-off shotgun. This is a chilling film that effectively shows the contradiction between the attractive outward demeanor of many psychopaths—even a young one as seen here—and their lack of internal anxiety or genuine concern for others.

Examination Items

IDENTIFICATION AND SHORT-ANSWER QUESTIONS
1. Define "moral insanity."
2. What are positive spikes among sociopaths?
3. What are the prominent characteristics of the paranoid personality disorder?

4. What is the histrionic personality disorder?
5. What is the narcissistic personality disorder?
6. What is the avoidant personality disorder?
7. What is the dependent personality disorder?
8. What is the compulsive personality disorder?
9. What is the passive-aggressive personality disorder?
10. What is the schizoid personality disorder?
11. What is the schizotypal personality disorder?
12. What is the borderline personality disorder?

ESSAY QUESTIONS
1. Discuss the criteria DSM-III-R requires to make a diagnosis of antisocial personality.
2. Discuss Cleckley's criteria for making a diagnosis of antisocial personality.
3. What is the experimental evidence that psychopaths are physiologically under-aroused?
4. Describe the Lykken, Schachter and Latane, and Schmauk studies of psychopaths, their results, and how they are usually interpreted.
5. What is the evidence for a genetic contribution to the antisocial personality?

CHAPTER 16

Childhood Disorders and Mental Retardation

Overview

The disorders and topics in this chapter are interesing in their own right, but they also highlight critical dimensions to all psychopathology, such as the difficulties of accounting for situational and developmental factors. They also emphasize the combination of biological and experiental factors that produce most forms of abnormality. Although some students may have little initial interest in the childhood disorders, others will have a passionate interest, and a few will have shown some of these disorders when younger or have a family member who exhibits them. A major objective is to educate all students for their eventual role as parents, as well as to prepare those bound for careers in education or psychology for advanced coursework.

Although this chapter is a brief survey of the childhood disorders, the content can fit comfortably into a single class meeting. More time can well be spent if desired, but most instructors will have little flexibility by this time in the term and will need to treat this topic sparingly to allow time for tying the course content together at the end and for considering the important social issues raised in Chapters 18 and 19. The text presents the basic childhood topics clearly, and the sample lecture outline assumes the text will be used to present most of the specific information.

Sample Lecture Outline

1. Begin by saying, "The text states that the problems of childhood and adolescence are more difficult to understand than the problems of adults." Why is this believed to be the case and do you personally agree with this position? Use the resulting discussion to help students appreciate the issues raised in the book, as well as to mention others that may occur to them. The special difficulties posed by childhood disorders are stressed in this chapter and need emphasis at the outset.

2. Mention the diversity of classification systems for childhood disorders. List the major disruptive, emotional, habit and eating, developmental, and gender identity disorders, but do not attempt to touch on each specific disorder in detail. Focus instead on those of special interest to you or the class (the popular topics of autism or anorexia nervosa and bulimia, for example). The general issues around prediction and treatment are more important in an introductory course than any of the specific problems.

3. Discuss treatment briefly, including the psychodynamic and behavioral methods used for the various disorders. Emphasize that the biomedical model and the whole notion of "treatment" makes less sense for many of the childhood disorders than do educational approaches designed to facilitate learning and normal developmental processes.

4. Before concluding the discussion of childhood disorders, emphasize the incidence figures for the problems presented in the text and the implications of these data for prevention. Point out that for clinicians committed to preventing problems in adults, the most potentially valuable direction when significant problems appear is to promote effective parenting, education, and treatment of children.

Demonstrations

1. Arrange a field trip to a mental retardation center, day-care program for children with developmental disabilities, or a sheltered workshop. Residential and outpatient treatment programs for emotionally disturbed children are unlikely to allow student tours, but those working with retarded populations may be eager to have your class visit. Visits such as these will do much to give students a realistic feel for children they may never have seen or thought seriously about when growing up.

2. Another option is to arrange a visit to a day-care center for three- and four-year-olds. Suggest students spend an hour or two observing and playing with the children and then lead a discussion afterwards on what they saw. Ask them to apply the criteria they read about in the text to their observations and to ask what, if anything, they observed that they would consider abnormal. This exercise will make clear the necessity of using developmental expectancies when judging childhood behavior.

3. Have students list their childhood phobias on pieces of paper and tabulate them on the board. Encourage students to discuss the things that used to frighten them and how the fears became of less concern or went away altogether—if they did!

Supplemental Readings

Dawson, G., & Mesibov, G. (1983). Childhood psychosis. In E. Walker & M. Roberts, *Handbook of clinical child psychology*. New York: Wiley. This is an excellent general overview of childhood psychotic disorders, going into much more detail than the text. Autism and childhood schizophrenia are both covered.

DeMyer, M., Hingtgen, J. N., & Jackson, R. (1981). Infantile autism reviewed: A decade of research. *Schizophrenia Bulletin, 7,* 388–451. This article surveys and critically evaluates research on autism, especially research on communication deficit models.

Films

Select films on childhood disorders with caution. Most old films are based on discredited views, such as Bettelheim's views on the psychogenic causes of autism, or they advocate psychodynamically oriented insight therapy for mild problems such as school phobia, stuttering, or enuresis, although behavioral techniques have been shown to be superior.

David: A portrait of a retarded youth (28 minutes, Filmmakers Library, Inc., 133 E. 58th St., New York, NY 10022) is an award-winning portrait of a seventeen-year-old young man with Down's syndrome who has just finished playing a retarded man in a film about mongolism based on his life. David seems to have loved being in the drama and talks freely about other setbacks and triumphs in his life. This is an inspiring and uplifting film.

One of our own (16 minutes, Filmmakers Library, Inc., 133 E. 58th St., New York, NY 10022). This film is about the life of David MacFarlane, the young man interviewed in the *David* film above. This film has more of a story than *David* and makes a nice companion to that character sketch.

Examination Items

IDENTIFICATION AND SHORT-ANSWER QUESTIONS

1. What are conduct disorders?
2. What is an attention-deficit hyperactivity disorder?
3. What is Achievement Place and what evidence suggests it is effective?
4. What kind of drug therapy is effective for hyperactive children?
5. How do phobias of children differ from those of adults?
6. What is school phobia?

7. What is enuresis?
8. Describe delayed feedback, shadowing, and syllable-timed speech as treatments for stuttering.
9. What is anorexia nervosa and how is it different from bulimia?
10. What is the set-point hypothesis?
11. What is the cause of cultural-familial retardation?
12. What is Down's syndrome?
13. What causes phenylketonuria (PKU)?
14. Differentiate specific and pervasive developmental difficulties.
15. What is echolalia?
16. What are pronominal reversals?

ESSAY QUESTIONS
1. Why are the problems of childhood more difficult to describe and define than the problems of adulthood?
2. Discuss various theories and research findings on the possible origins of conduct disorders.
3. Differentiate mild, moderate, severe, and profound levels of mental retardation.
4. Describe the symptoms of autism and the most commonly accepted position at present about what causes this disorder.

CHAPTER 17

Disorders of the Nervous System and Psychopathology

Overview

Compared to most abnormal psychology texts, the treatment of the organic disorders in this chapter takes an unusual and ambitious approach. Instead of surveying the many forms of psychopathology known to have an organic basis, the importance of neurology to the study of psychopathology is emphasized. The structural and functional organization of the nervous system and general aspects of neurological disorders are covered in detail.

Although this chapter is challenging and of excellent quality, many students are likely to find it of less personal interest and relevance than previous chapters on more psychologically caused disorders. In part this is because this chapter is more of an up-to-date overview of neuroscience than a description of various organically based forms of psychopathology and in part because most undergraduates have less interest in psychological disorders resulting from biology, which are seen as untreatable with psychological methods. This means that instructors will need to emphasize the relevance and importance of the neurological information that is presented. A good way to create a positive set beforehand is to warn students that although they may find the material in Chapter 17 initially challenging and of less interest than some of the other disorders, they will eventually see this as one of the most important chapters in the text.

Because of differences among instructors in knowledge and enthusiasm for neuroscience, they will vary in how much emphasis they give the anatomical and physiological details presented in the text and in how fully they require students to master these details. Some instructors may expect students to have only a general understanding; others will expect most details to be learned as well.

A reasonable option for most instructors is to spend one class on neurological background information, on the anatomy and workings of the brain, and a second class on specific organic disorders. The class on specific disorders can be supplemented by including descriptions of other disorders not mentioned or touched on only briefly in the text. If only a single class can be devoted to this chapter, focus on a combination of general principles and specific disorders. Regardless of what approach is taken, instructors should emphasize the final section, which puts organically based disorders into perspective. The sample outline that follows takes the first option and assumes two classes will be used.

Sample Lecture Outline

Move at a slower pace than usual in this class to be sure students have ample time to ask for clarification. Cover the important points and try to offset the tendency of many students to see these concepts as facts to memorize rather than to understand.

1. Begin with an introductory note stressing *why* these neurological processes are so important to understanding many forms of psychopathology. Emphasize that some disorders can be accounted for totally by structure and function and that others result solely from experience. If you can help students experience a sense of awe at the complexity of the nervous system and the intellectual satisfaction of complex neurological problem solving, they are more likely to find this chapter relevant and important, both for the potential of the biomedical model to expand our knowledge of psychopathology and of various forms of psychopathology to expand our understanding of the brain.

2. Following the organization in the text, focus on the various levels of nervous system organization and their effects on psychopathology. Synapses and biochemical variables have already been covered elsewhere, but the topics of supportive tissue, front-back, horizontal, and vertical organization, the critical balance of inhibition and excitation, redundancy, recovery, and vulnerability need brief attention. Emphasize that, taken as a group, these offer a complex model of nervous system function that accounts for much that is known about neuropathology.

3. Bring this class to a close by touching on the general aspects of nervous system diseases. Differentiate the effects of localized versus widespread damage, excitatory versus inhibitory dysfunction, deficits in Luria's three domains of higher brain functions, and the techniques used to diagnose neurological disorders.

4. Begin the second class with an overview of the kind of organic problems that can create significant deficits in mental functioning and independent living. The text touches only briefly on the difference between acute and chronic organic brain syndromes, problems resulting from tumors, and the senile dementias, and you may want to go into more depth here. Emphasize that correctly diagnosing the cause of these disorders requires complex problem-solving, in addition to detailed knowledge of neuroanatomy and neurophysiology.

5. Present a case illustrating the personal distress commonly experienced by individuals suffering from any of the aphasias. If students can empathize with such persons and imagine how *they* would feel if unable to use language normally, they will be much more likely to find these disorders engaging.

6. Spend most of the class on the amnesias, differentiating the varied factors that can lead to memory loss. Be sure students appreciate the different theories of memory and memory loss and how the theory proposed by the authors has advantages over previous formulations, especially regarding retrograde amnesia.

7. Before leaving the organic disorders, say a few words about treatment. Students tend to view these problems pessimistically, assuming that psychotherapy is irrelevant because the causes of the problems are organic. Stress that a great deal can be done to reduce the added stress resulting from individuals' *psychological reactions* to their disability and that even the problems of the aged are not as hopeless as is commonly believed. If students can leave this topic with renewed awe at the wonder of the human brain and nervous system and an image of organically afflicted individuals as still human, a major objective will have been met.

Demonstrations

1. Pass around copies of geometric figures (similar to those on the Bender-Gestalt or Graham-Kendell Memory For Designs tests) and ask students to copy them as closely as they can. Then show samples of the kind of drawings typically obtained from populations suffering from organic syndromes. This demonstration will emphasize for students how abilities we take for granted are a product of complex neurofunctions.

2. Encourage students to spend an hour or so visiting a nursing home and talking with the patients. They will be sure to observe some of the emotional and intellectual deficits characterizing many organically damaged persons.

Supplemental Readings

Gardner, H. (1975). *The shattered mind: The person after brain damage.* New York: Knopf. This introduction to brain damage provides excellent background information and rich case studies that can be used to supplement lectures. This book is written at an appropriate level for abnormal psychology students, and selected parts can also be assigned as supplemental reading.

Sacks, O. (1987). *The man who mistook his wife for a hat and other clinical tales.* New York: Harper & Row. As already cited under Chapter 3, this collection provides useful clinical illustrations for presentation here.

Scientific American. (1970). *The brain.* San Francisco: Freeman. This is a collection of *Scientific American* articles about neuroanatomy, neurochemistry, neurophysiology, and physiological psychology. All are written by prominent brain scientists in a nontechnical, easily understandable style.

Springer, S. P., & Deutsch, G. (1981). *Left brain, right brain.* San Francisco: Freeman. This is a general coverage of what is currently known about cerebral hemisphere functions, and it will answer most questions you or your students will have about this topic.

Films

The brain and behavior (22 minutes, McGraw-Hill Textfilms, 110 15th St., Del Mar, CA 92014). This film shows two different approaches to studying the functions of different brain parts. Studies of brain-damaged individuals are presented, and research on brain stimulation studies is summarized.

The hidden universe: The brain (48 minutes, McGraw-Hill Textfilms, 110 15th St., Del Mar, CA 92014). This film presents an overview of brain functioning, including issues such as perception, memory, and brain disorders.

Organic reaction—Senile type (10 minutes, McGraw-Hill Textfilms, 110 15th St., Del Mar, CA 92014). This is from the McGraw-Hill "Mental Symptoms" series and demonstrates the common symptoms of senility.

Examination Items

IDENTIFICATION AND SHORT-ANSWER QUESTIONS
1. Differentiate between gray and white matter.
2. What is disinhibition?
3. Differentiate phonological and deep dyslexia.
4. What is redundancy in the nervous system?
5. Why can there be recovery of function after damage to the nervous system?
6. Describe the vulnerability of neurosystems.
7. What are Luria's divisions of higher brain functions?
8. How do CAT scans, MRI's, and PET scans produce visual images of the brain?
9. Differentiate expressive and receptive aphasia.
10. What is an apraxia?
11. What is perseveration?
12. How are Alzheimer's disease and Pick's disease similar and different?
13. Differentiate explicit and implicit tests of memory.
14. Differentiate anterograde and retrograde amnesia.
15. Differentiate the consolidation block and retrieval theories of amnesia.

ESSAY QUESTIONS

1. Discuss one of the three ways of viewing the organization of the nervous system, indicating how damage at various locations is likely to be revealed.
2. What are the general strategies and specific techniques used in making neurological diagnoses?
3. What are the basic features of the amnesic syndrome?

The Law and Politics of Abnormality

Overview

This is an excellent chapter to begin pulling the course together for closure. It raises critical social issues surrounding psychopathology, especially how the legal safeguards enjoyed by citizens in democratic republics are stretched and abused in the name of protection, both of the individual and of the state. More than any other single chapter, Chapter 18 is important to the education of students as citizens. It can help them become informed about the ways the mentally troubled have been treated in the past in the name of treatment and can sensitize them to the continuing need to balance civil liberties with effective and humane treatment.

The content of Chapter 18 lends itself well to discussion and debate among students. The sample lecture outline and suggested demonstrations take advantage of this. Although there are fewer specific concepts to be covered here, the general principles presented are both important and complex, well worth coverage in class. Avoid the temptation to delete this chapter if time is rushed at the end. Students will be quite interested in the material—outraged by many of the abuses cited—and will need to examine their attitudes and emotional reactions and to understand well the legal principles presented.

The sample outline assumes a single class is devoted to this chapter, but, if available, an additional one can be spent in extended discussion or on some of the suggested demonstrations.

Sample Lecture Outline

1. Begin with an introduction to the legal and social issues to be covered. Encourage students to view the cases and legal qualifications as useful "exceptions that prove the rule" about the way our society guarantees freedom and rights to its citizens in actuality. Point out that much as psycho-

pathology can teach us much about brain function, the social context of psychopathology can also teach much about civil rights in our society.

2. Focus first on involuntary commitment. Ask students to share their opinion about whether the individuals in the brief examples given in the text should or should not be confined against their will. If so, why and for how long? Most students will have no concrete idea of what is required in your state to commit someone. Present the local procedures and criteria, contrasting them with those discussed in the text (impaired judgment, need for treatment, dangerousness to others, dangerousness to self, and grave disability). To stimulate discussion, ask how likely they would be to use the local commitment procedures if a relative were planning to sell her house, marry someone she had met just last week, and head for South America aboard a tramp steamer. Ask if their feelings would differ if the person announcing these plans was their brother, sister, father, or mother.

The section in the text on how the three *standards of proof* commonly used in American courts have been applied to cases of commitment is especially important and illuminating. Be certain that students appreciate that legal decisions about anything are always made under some such guidelines and that the current standard for commitment is a relatively recent and very appropriate compromise between what is common in civil and criminal courts.

3. Students will have much misinformation about the insanity defense. It is important that they be able to clearly differentiate between the three common tests used in making this defense; classroom demonstration 1 gives situations for the class to judge. Whether or not the demonstration is used, spend some time comparing the M'Naghten, Durham, and ALI rules. Be certain students appreciate that the rare occurrence of winning a criminal case using an insanity defense is frequently not in the accused's best interests, given the lack of due process and poor conditions common in hospitals for the "criminally insane." Discuss the contradictions of the new "guilty but mentally ill" verdict.

4. Bring this class to a close by asking, "When does the state have an obligation to protect the public and disturbed individuals by limiting their freedom when they act contrary to common practice?" Many campus communities have visible "street people" or eccentrics. Whenever possible, personalize the issues by asking students to apply their arguments to these individuals. Help them see that even when most students would agree that intervention is appropriate, the difficult business of judging risk and likely cause in a given case remains.

Demonstrations

1. Read the following cases to the class and ask them to apply the M'Naghten, Durham, and ALI tests to determine if the individuals in each case qualify for a verdict of "not guilty by reason of insanity."

a. Jed Hough, a sixty-five-year-old resident of an isolated cove in the West Virginia mountains, is a devout believer in fundamental Christianity. To him the world is the battlefield between the devil and Jesus Christ, and the righteous can never let down their guard lest Satan "git hold of their immortal souls." Jed was particularly upset one night after attending a hearing of the local school board during which the biology curriculum and certain controversial novels were the subject of much heated and, frankly, ignorant discussion. Soon after returning home, Jed began a lengthy prayer session that was interrupted about 10:30 P.M. by a newspaper reporter's knock at the door. Jed saw the man's out-of-state car out the front room window and knew "this mustta been one'a Satan's boys, like what God had told me to watch out fer." Jed reports he instantly knew what he had to do and without a moment's reflection, he got his shotgun down from off the wall and fired both barrels through the front door, mortally wounding the reporter.

b. Gilbert Jarret is a twenty-four-year-old college senior who was arrested for exposing his genitalia in the lobby of a women's dormitory at a neighboring college. He had a long-standing history of exhibitionism and was in therapy at the time of this most recent incident. He has never touched the women involved, never exposed himself to children, and has done so only after fighting the strong urge to do so for as long as he can—usually at least several hours, sometimes days. He clearly suffers from a chronic and intransigent case of exhibitionism.

c. Donna Harding was first molested sexually by her father when she was eleven years old. She was always a "prim and proper little girl" and was as much afraid others would find out what her father had done to her as angry at her father. Mr. Harding had regular sexual intercourse with her—usually once a week—until Donna left home to go to college at age eighteen. During her first semester, she found herself increasingly anxious when on dates with boys, eventually refusing to accept invitations from them at all. By the spring of her freshman year, she had become withdrawn with girl friends as well, so much so that her roommate asked to move in with another girl. Because of her reclusiveness and suspicions, she was referred for treatment by the dormitory counselor to the university psychological clinic, where she was diagnosed as a paranoid schizophrenic, given anti-psychotic medications, and seen on an outpatient basis. Her symptoms gradually improved, and she was able to complete most of her spring classes successfully, although at far below her usually high level of academic performance. Two weeks after she returned home for the summer, her father approached her sexually one evening when her mother was out of the house. She told him to get into bed to wait for her and calmly walked to the den, where she took down his deer rifle, loaded it, and returned to empty the magazine into his chest.

2. Ask student volunteers to seek out a bizarre street person or two in your community. Instruct the students to find out why the people live as they do and how they would feel if forced to live in a hospital, halfway house, or other structured "treatment" setting. Even if no one is willing to speak to the students, they will learn a lot about such unusual-appearing persons. If students succeed in completing an interview, allow them time to report back to the class on their experiences as a stimulus for discussion of the issues presented in this chapter.

3. Ask students to divide into two teams to do background research for a class debate on whether David Berkowitz, the "Son of Sam" killer in the New York City area a few years ago should have been allowed to stand trial. Two psychiatrists ruled he was *not* competent to stand trial, but the judge ruled in favor of a third who argued he was competent. Suggest students consult newspaper files from the period for evidence to be used to argue both sides of this issue. Have a few students remain uninvolved and serve as a jury for the proceedings. (David Abrahamsen's article, Unmasking Son of Sam's demons, *The New York Times Magazine*, July 1, 1979, 20–22, summarizes the evidence if you wish to present this case yourself or to save students the labor of researching newspaper files.)

Supplemental Reading

Oran, D. (1973, August). Judges and psychiatrists lock up too many people. *Psychology Today*, 20–28. The author uses many case examples to support his thesis that institutionalization for treatment is an overused and ineffective response of society to many forms of deviant behavior. It frequently is at odds with the rights of institutionalized mental patients to due process as well as appropriate treatment.

Schwitzgebel, K. (1975). A contractual model for the protection of the rights of mental patients. *American Psychologist, 30,* 815–820. The author criticizes the traditional medical treatment approach to protecting patients' rights and proposes an alternative means of achieving this goal which conceptualizes patient treatment as a contractual activity in which both parties know what to expect, have a reasonable chance of getting what they want, and are able to sue if they are not pleased with the outcome.

Films

Titticut Follies (85 minutes, Grove Press, 5589 New Peachtree Rd., Atlanta, GA 30341). This is an award-winning film about the treatment given patients at a prison for the criminally insane. The film takes its name from a show the patients put on for the amusement of their guards. Graphic, at times shocking, this film is certain to impress students with the inhumanity shown at times to relatively powerless psychiatric patients.

Examination Items

IDENTIFICATION AND SHORT-ANSWER QUESTIONS

1. What was "Operation Baxtrom"?
2. What does it mean to say someone's behavior and choices about living have been "psychiatrized"?
3. What is the "Patients' Bill of Rights"?
4. What is the M'Naghten rule?
5. What is the Durham rule?
6. What is the ALI rule?

ESSAY QUESTIONS

1. Discuss the conditions commonly used to judge an individual as being in need of psychiatric treatment against his or her will.
2. Differentiate the following legal standards of proof and how they are applied to psychological disorders: preponderance of evidence, beyond a reasonable doubt, and clear and convincing proof.
3. Discuss the three rules for the insanity defense and give examples of cases that might pass one rule but would fail to pass others.
4. What is the "Guilty but mentally ill verdict"? How is it different from other rules, and what are its limitations?

A Consumer's Guide to Psychological Treatment

Overview

This is an ideal chapter to bring the text and the course to a close. Not only is treatment of high personal relevance and interest to students, this last chapter provides an excellent vehicle to tie together many themes and concepts that have been discussed before. Students may still entertain myths about therapy and therapists, and this is a good place to address these topics directly. It also gives them a chance to ask questions of more personal concern: the questions they had before beginning the course, as well as those stimulated by what they have learned. Like the previous chapter on legal issues, Chapter 19 lends itself well to discussion and demonstration.

A valuable objective here is for students to be able to select the best therapeutic intervention for a variety of specific and general psychological problems. Although the chapters on specific theoretical perspectives and diagnostic categories presented data on treatment effectiveness, this information has not been brought together in one section until now. The sample lecture outline recommends reviewing treatment by describing specific problems and asking students which treatments they would recommend, and why they propose the ones they do.

When planning the class session(s) for this chapter, include some time for students to reflect on the entire course, on what, among the many things they have learned, most stands out and on what the study of abnormal psychology has taught them about human nature. Although the class atmosphere during discussion in final classes is commonly slower and more reflective than previously, the combination of intellectual, attitudinal, and interpersonal objectives that are met makes it an excellent way to bring a memorable course to a close.

Sample Lecture Outline

This lecture outline heavily emphasizes discussion. Following it completely will take two classes. If only one session is available, include fewer topics and less discussion.

1. Begin by indicating that many forms of psychotherapy will be put into perspective in this session for the purpose of tying together what students have been learning throughout the course about treatment. Also indicate that the chapter will help them become better-informed consumers about therapy and therapists, given that many class members will one day seek therapy for themselves or a family member.

2. Proceed by presenting the following list of statements and asking students to write down (using a seven-point scale) how much they agree with them:

a. Different forms of psychotherapy work in different ways, and these differences account for most of their effectiveness.

b. Although its high cost and the scarcity of trained analysts makes it unavailable to everyone, psychoanalysis is still the best form of psychotherapy.

c. Behavior therapy is mainly useful with extreme forms of psycho-pathology and with patients with whom it is difficult to do "talking psychotherapy" effectively.

d. Psychotropic drugs should be given to mental patients only when nothing else will work because the drugs distort their conscious experience and reduce their ability to relate to others and to understand and control their own thoughts, feelings, and lives.

e. To be effective, psychotherapists must make their patients so uncomfortable that the patients will be motivated to change.

Plot the distributions of students' scores on the board before saying that there is considerable evidence that each of the statements is generally *false*. Give students an opportunity to react to and discuss their ratings of these statements, but do not spend a great deal of time on them unless you wish to use extended discussion of them to focus on the topics raised in the chapter.

3. Say a few words about the different professional groups doing psychotherapy. Most students will understand the distinctions made in the text on their own, but be certain they appreciate that all legitimate practitioners have done several years of postgraduate work involving supervised practicum or internship experience. Point out that there is considerable variability in the technical skill shown *within* each professional group and avoid critical generalizations about practitioners with other than your own type of professional training (remember that some students may have parents who are members of any group you may malign). Although this is not a good place to fight professional battles, commenting on such tensions may help students decide which, if any, mental health career to pursue.

4. Whether you lecture or use discussion, emphasize the common ingredients of psychotherapy, pointing out how these cut across all forms of psychotherapy and account for much of their effectiveness. To use discussion ask, "What factors about therapists and therapy are necessary for the therapy to be effective?" Either way, emphasize that although these general effects are necessary, they are not sufficient.

5. Avoid going into the specific forms of therapy described. They have been mentioned before, and it is more important for students to review and apply this knowledge than to have it repeated. Instead, ask students to request clarification and to give their personal evaluations of the various forms available. For example, ask, "If you suddenly won a 'therapy sweepstakes' and could receive from a master therapist of that school any form of psychotherapy you wished for up to six months, which would you choose, and why?"

6. To help students integrate their knowledge of therapies and diagnostic categories, ask them to recommend various treatments for several specific problems. For example, ask what therapy they would recommend for someone requesting therapy for:

    a. fear about going outside the house
    b. repetitive thoughts that they were going to kill their children and elaborate household cleaning rituals
    c. vague feelings that life had lost its meaning and no longer made any sense
    d. the feeling that others were able to read their thoughts and control their actions
    e. a drinking problem that had destroyed their family and career
    f. depression that was not so severe that the person could not perform everyday tasks, but that made living a dull, energyless, and unrewarding experience
    g. depression so severe the person was considering suicide and was unable to go to work
    h. an aversion to eating and the feeling they were fat, even though everyone told them they were becoming too thin
    i. a problem ejaculating too quickly when having sexual intercourse
    j. a compulsion, especially strong when tired, to steal women's undergarments from lingerie shops

This exercise will take at least fifteen minutes, but it can easily be expanded to consume much of a class session if more details are asked for and if more students are encouraged to participate in the discussion.

7. Bring this chapter to a close by commenting on the efforts to actively seek high-risk individuals and to provide them with supportive or educational interventions to prevent psychopathology. Point out that prevention

is a worthy goal for the future that is tied up with the structure of society. Mention how society's institutions can aid or interfere with optimal human development.

Demonstrations

1. Ask student volunteers to simulate an individual with an emotional problem unknown to you and to do a short role play illustrating how various psychodynamic, cognitive, or behavioral psychotherapists would interview the individual. These need not be lengthy simulations. It is better to do several short simulations than a single lengthy one. This also gives more students an opportunity to participate as pseudopatients. An alternative is to let students role play the therapist as well, behaving as they believe the different therapists might act. Either way, allow a few minutes for the class to react to and comment on the demonstration.

2. Ask student volunteers to seek out in groups of three various practitioners in your community and interview them on how, in actual practice, they do therapy. Have the students present what they learned in class for common discussion. What they are likely to learn is that there is far more variety and eclecticism among practicing clinicians than textbooks would suggest.

Supplemental Readings

American Journal of Community Psychology. The June, 1982, special issue presents summaries of eight programs identified by Emory Cowen as having experimentally demonstrated preventive effectiveness. The programs are focused toward a wide variety of problems and ages. For example, programs are described and evaluated which aim to offer support or specific training in needed interpersonal skills for the newly separated, students beginning high school, juveniles at risk for abusing drugs, mothers on public assistance, the elderly, and preschool children.

Colby, K. (1951). *A primer for psychotherapists*. New York: Wiley-Interscience. This classic introduction to insight psychotherapy is still in print. It covers in a simple way all the questions beginning therapists have about what actually happens in therapy. Although typically assigned to first-year residents and graduate students, it would make good supplemental reading for interested students in this course as well.

Dohrenwend, B. S. (1978). Social stress and community psychology. *American Journal of Community Psychology, 6,* 1–14. Barbara Dohrenwend presents a model for preventive mental health in this article that differentiates individual preventive and treatment interventions and group and community-focused interventions. It offers an excellent overview of prevention and the community mental health movement. The reading is simple enough for motivated undergraduates.

Films

Three approaches to psychotherapy (Psychological Films, 110 N. Wheeler St., Orange, CA 92669). This is a classic comparison of Carl Rogers (48 minutes), Albert Ellis (36 minutes), and Fritz Perls (32 minutes). Even though these are old films, they are unique in their portrayal of three therapists interviewing the same patient, Gloria. Each film must be ordered separately, and each is an excellent example of these three famous psychotherapists' work. Color enhanced videotapes of this classic series are now available.

Examination Items

IDENTIFICATION AND SHORT-ANSWER QUESTIONS

1. Differentiate the professional training required to become a psychiatrist, a psychologist, and a psychiatric social worker.
2. What training is required to become a psychoanalyst?
3. What is the "therapeutic alliance"?
4. What is the placebo effect?
5. What are the therapist qualities of "empathy," "warmth," and "genuineness" and what is their contribution to effective psychotherapy?
6. What is resistance?
7. What broad categories of improvement are commonly used to evaluate treatment effectiveness?
8. What are containment services?
9. What is a hot-line?

ESSAY QUESTIONS

1. Discuss the common elements of all psychotherapy and how they are thought to contribute to effective treatment.
2. Compare and contrast therapies designed to treat specific problems and those to promote personal insight.
3. What efforts are being made to prevent psychopathology?